Exercise Testing and Prescription Lab Manual

Edmund O. Acevedo, PhD, FACSM

Michael A. Starks, MS, CSCS

Division of Exercise Science
The University of Mississippi

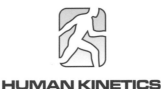

HUMAN KINETICS

ISBN: 0-7360-4694-1

Acquisitions Editor: Michael S. Bahrke, PhD; **Developmental Editor:** Elaine H. Mustain; **Assistant Editors:** Maggie Schwarzentraub, Derek Campbell, Susan C. Hagan, Ragen E. Sanner; **Copyeditor:** Barbara Juhas Walsh; **Proofreader:** Erin Cler; **Permission Manager:** Dalene Reeder; **Graphic Designer:** Robert Reuther; **Graphic Artist:** Yvonne Griffith; **Photo Manager;** Kareema McLendon; **Cover Designer:** Keith Blomberg; **Photographer (cover):** Edmund O. Acevedo; **Photographer (interior):** © Human Kinetics except where otherwise noted. Photos on pages 11, 35, 36, 77, 78, 80, 86, 88, © Edmund O. Acevedo; **Art Manager:** Kelly Hendren; **Illustrators:** Kelly Hendren and Mic Greenberg; **Printer:** United Graphics

Printed in the United States of America   10 9 8 7 6 5 4 3 2

Human Kinetics

Web site: www.HumanKinetics.com

United States: Human Kinetics, P.O. Box 5076, Champaign, IL 61825-5076
800-747-4457
e-mail: humank@hkusa.com

Canada: Human Kinetics, 475 Devonshire Road, Unit 100, Windsor, ON N8Y 2L5
800-465-7301 (in Canada only)
e-mail: orders@hkcanada.com

Europe: Human Kinetics, 107 Bradford Road, Stanningley
Leeds LS28 6AT, United Kingdom
+44 (0) 113 255 5665
e-mail: hk@hkeurope.com

Australia: Human Kinetics, 57A Price Avenue, Lower Mitcham, South Australia 5062
08 8277 1555
e-mail: liaw@hkaustralia.com

New Zealand: Human Kinetics, Division of Sports Distributors NZ Ltd.
P.O. Box 300 226 Albany, North Shore City, Auckland
0064 9 448 1207
e-mail: info@humankinetics.co.nz

To my wife and best friend, Tracy, and my children Eddie and Elena.

EOA

Contents

List of Tables

Preface

Evidence demonstrating the importance of physical fitness to enhanced quality of life and longevity has received much attention in the past 15 years. The health benefits of regular exercise are unquestioned. Furthermore, researchers have defined exercise guidelines that clarify the safest, most effective, and most efficient manner for participation in an exercise program. The association that has taken the lead in defining these guidelines and has established the gold standard for professional practice and certification in exercise testing and prescription is the American College of Sports Medicine (ACSM). ACSM has certified close to 20,000 individuals in the past 10 years. Of the five different levels of certification, the Health Fitness Instructor certification (HFI) has had the greatest number of participants. More than 12,000 people have been certified as Health Fitness Instructors in the past 10 years. This laboratory manual addresses the necessary skills and techniques for successful completion of the HFI certification.

A person certified as a Health Fitness Instructor is a professional qualified to assess, design, and implement fitness programs for apparently healthy people and for people with controlled disease. *ACSM's Guidelines for Exercise Testing and Prescription, Sixth Edition,* presents certification guidelines. A component of the requirements for each certification, including HFI, is a practical application of the knowledge and skills associated with exercise testing and prescription. The easy-to-follow, step-by-step experiential-based learning laboratories in this text correspond with the practical skills required for successful completion of the HFI certification exam. Furthermore, the *Exercise Testing and Prescription Lab Manual* is an excellent supplement to undergraduate courses designed to prepare students to take the ACSM Health Fitness Instructor examination.

This laboratory manual contains three sections:

- Pretest responsibilities
- Exercise-testing techniques
- Exercise prescription

The first section includes three labs that focus on the HFI's responsibilities in advance of performing an exercise test. These labs present information pertaining to safety procedures, requirements for exercise-testing equipment, calibration of equipment, medical history evaluation, risk factor evaluation and stratification, and informed consent. Case studies direct significant attention toward risk factor evaluation and stratification.

The second section includes five labs that focus on the techniques used to assess the components of health-related fitness (cardiorespiratory function, body composition, muscular strength and endurance, and flexibility). An additional lab in this section presents information on electrocardiogram (ECG) placement and operating ECG equipment. The application procedures in these labs include step-by-step instructions, data collection worksheets, diagrams depicting appropriate techniques, and charts that present norms for making comparisons by age and gender.

The final section of the *Exercise Testing and Prescription Lab Manual* focuses on exercise prescription. The initial lab in this section addresses the calculation of metabolic work for use in exercise prescription. The next two labs focus on the three phases of exercise prescription (initial, improvement, and maintenance), assessment of a participant's goals, and gaining the participant's commitment to the exercise prescription. The final lab in this manual challenges students to apply the techniques and principles presented in the laboratory manual by developing case studies. Appendix C provides a summary of the effects of common pharmacological agents on cardiorespiratory responses at rest and during exercise, appendix D contains common metric conversions used in exercise testing and prescription calculations, and appendix E offers a list of metabolic and anthropometric formulas.

Each lab features an easy-to-follow format including the headings "Purpose," "Materials," "Background Information," "Procedures," "Discussion Questions," and "References." The background section provides a framework for that lab but does not necessarily present all the knowledge required for an understanding of the rationale, theory, and physiological principles of the topics presented in that lab. The expectation is that more in-depth knowledge will be presented in a course lecture format or that students will research topics further to be able to answer any discussion questions they do not understand. In the procedures section, students will find all of the procedural information required to complete that lab. Many of the labs require data collection. To facilitate this process, this laboratory manual contains all the forms and worksheets that students will need to complete the lab assignments and collect the data in an organized manner. These forms, which may be photocopied by students who have purchased this manual, are located in appendix A and the worksheets in appendix B. Each lab identifies how many copies of which forms are needed to complete it so that students can bring enough copies of the appropriate forms and worksheets to that lab. Once the students who have purchased the manual become practioners, they may also copy forms from appendixes A and B for use with their clients. A glossary defines terms appearing in the text and appendixes.

This manual is organized in such a way as to take the reader progressively through each phase of exercise testing and prescription. In addition, the practical experiences that it provides for students reinforce specific information for the student or practitioner preparing for the HFI certification exam. Furthermore, these practical experiences are intended to complement a lecture course that presents to the student the knowledge base required for HFI certification. With its focused presentation of the skills included in the HFI certification exam, this manual fills a void for the health fitness practitioner studying for HFI certification.

Acknowledgments

This laboratory manual has been in development for 12 years, since the first author began teaching a course designed to instruct students in the application of exercise-testing techniques and exercise prescription. Throughout this period a number of colleagues have provided critical feedback that has enhanced the presentation of this manual. We would like to acknowledge those people. For their input and critical review of the laboratories during the initial stages of development, we thank Drs. Michael Meyers and Robert Kraemer. We would also like to acknowledge the work of Terry Garner, Naomi Howard, and Jason VanGotten, who, while completing their graduate assistantship responsibilities, greatly enhanced the presentation of these labs. Finally, the first author would like to express his appreciation to his wife, Tracy Acevedo, for her editorial expertise and support.

PART I

Pretest Responsibilities

PART I comprises three labs that focus on the HFI's responsibilities before performing an exercise test. These labs present information pertaining to safety procedures, requirements for exercise-testing equipment, calibration of equipment, medical history evaluation, risk factor evaluation and stratification, and informed consent. Case studies direct significant attention toward risk factor evaluation and stratification.

Orientation to Lab Instruments, Procedures, and Responsibilities

PURPOSE

This lab accomplishes the following: It demonstrates to and familiarizes students with the safety procedures, lab equipment, and instruments that they will use during labs throughout the course. It explains the procedures, requirements, and responsibilities for lab assignments.

MATERIALS

1. Cycle ergometer (e.g., Monark, Tunturi)
2. 12-lead electrocardiograph (ECG) (electrodes and cables)
3. 3-lead ECG telemetry system (electrodes and transmitters)
4. Treadmill
5. Rating of perceived exertion (RPE) scale (figure 5.2)
6. Flexibility-assessment devices (goniometer, sit-and-reach box, meter stick or yardstick, etc.)

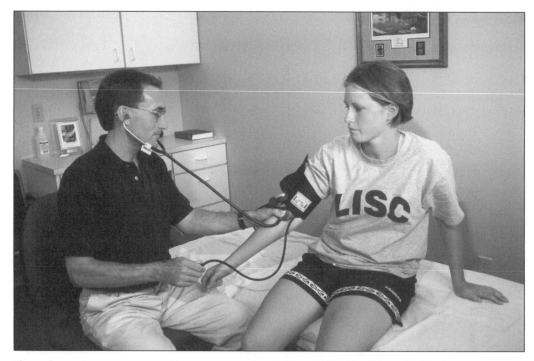

If you hope to assess your clients accurately and prescribe intelligently for them, you must begin by getting the kind of hands-on experience with testing equipment that this lab manual will provide.

7. Mercurial and aneroid sphygmomanometer
8. Stethoscope
9. Hand dynamometer
10. Barometer and thermometer
11. Scale and stadiometer
12. Body composition assessment devices

Procedures

1. The lab instructor describes preliminary preparation for exercise testing. The fitness instructor should be familiar with the following elements that are crucial to a safe, professional exercise-testing environment. The lab instructor will discuss each of these elements.

   a. Establishing emergency procedures
   b. Periodically practicing emergency drills
   c. Clearly posting emergency phone numbers
   d. Ensuring current CPR certification

  e. Maintaining an appropriately professional (clean, quiet, visually appealing) environment for testing

  f. Establishing policies to ensure adequate client privacy

  g. Checking and calibrating equipment frequently

2. Discuss the procedures and grading system.

3. The lab instructor briefly introduces and describes the items listed under "Materials." Students will practice using this equipment as they participate in the labs that follow in this course.

4. Review the units of the metric system (appendix D).

General Laboratory Instructions

1. Before each scheduled lab, read the instructions to become familiar with the materials you will use and the procedure you will follow.

2. The lab instructor will give additional verbal clarification and demonstrations when necessary. Listen and take notes as applicable.

3. You will usually work in groups of three or four. Organize your group quickly, selecting a recorder, a subject, and a technician. Become familiar with the responsibilities that each position entails. Rotate assignments during each lab if data is to be collected from more than one subject. (Note: Obtain data from all group members when possible.)

4. One member of the group should be responsible for obtaining the equipment needed for the day, maintaining it accordingly during the work period, and returning it after the lab period. Be extremely careful with all equipment, because it is very expensive and difficult to replace. Return all equipment to the exact place from which it was taken, and be sure that it is clean and that the storage facility remains well organized.

5. The recorder should record the observations immediately as they are taken. Record only raw data; perform any calculations and conversions after the data are collected.

6. Work seriously and quietly. Noise may disrupt the subject or interfere with accurate reporting of the results. If basal rates are to be established or if blood pressures are to be recorded, eliminate all noise.

7. Listen to final instructions. Do not leave the lab before checking with the lab instructor.

8. Appropriate clothing (shorts, T-shirt, sweats, athletic shoes, and socks) is required. In addition, you will need a calculator for computation of data.

9. Complete lab assignments, including discussion questions, after each lab meeting. Type the labs and hand them in before the next scheduled lab begins.

Calibrating Lab Instruments

PURPOSE

This lab demonstrates how to calibrate equipment for exercise testing and prescription and why such calibration is important.

MATERIALS

1. Cycle ergometer
2. Sphygmomanometers
3. Weight scales
4. Chatillon Scale/load cells
5. One copy of the Cycle Ergometer Calibration Worksheet (page 132)
6. One copy of the Sphygmomanometer/Aneroid Gauge Calibration Worksheet (page 133)
7. One copy of the Weight Scale Calibration Worksheet (page 134)
8. One copy of the Chatillon Scale/Load Cell Worksheet (page 135)

Background Information

Inaccurate instruments will introduce error into any procedure in which they are used. The process of adjusting or correcting an instrument to coincide with a known standard is referred to as *calibration*. Calibration is essential to reliable and valid data.

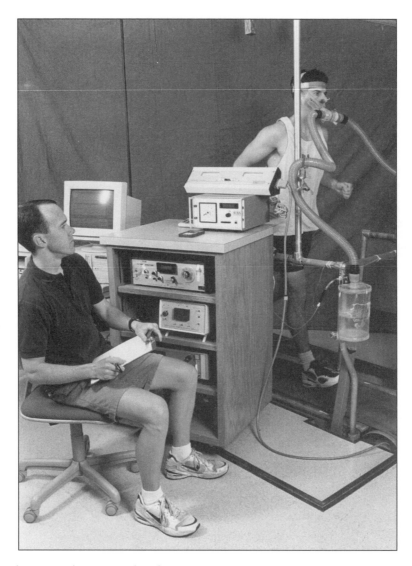

No matter how simple or complex the equipment you use, if it is not properly calibrated, it will not provide reliable or valid data.

In the simplest case, two scales of measurement might be compared against each other—for example, if we lay a meter stick alongside some reference measure, we can then compare the lengths and subdivisions of the two. Of course, in this case, to correct any error we might have to sand off the existing markings on the meter stick and etch new ones along the entire scale.

A reference quantity that has been previously determined to be within an acceptably small degree of error can be used as a calibration standard (reference measure). For example, a set of brass weight standards might be used to calibrate a balance scale for accurate weighing. In the case of a sophisticated electronic balance, adjustments can be made to reconcile small deviations of measurement from known weights. Some instruments, however, have no simple means of adjustment.

Error

There are two kinds of measurement errors, *random errors* and *systematic errors*. Random errors occur in all measurement, but good technique and consistency of methods can minimize them. You can estimate the degree of random error by performing repeated measurements on the same quantity with the same instrument and expressing the variability of the measurement with some statistic (i.e., standard error). Systematic errors arise when an instrument or procedure consistently overestimates or underestimates the quantities being measured.

The errors estimated in laboratory work are generally random errors. If a systematic error is detected, adjust the instrument (or procedure) to eliminate it.

Calibration Points

Consider the calibration of a hand dynamometer, which measures the strength of a person's handgrip. To check it for accuracy, you might secure its base to a supporting framework and suspend 50 kg of mass from its stirrup. Under these conditions, the pointer should be aligned with the 50 kg readout display. This procedure, however, would establish only whether the dial correctly indicates the acceleration of gravity on a mass of 50 kg. To be certain of the accuracy of the instrument throughout the range of its scale readings, you would need to check every distinguishable point within this range. Such a procedure is not generally practical. A reasonable compromise is to check several calibration points centered at about the middle of the expected range as well as several points at about the lowest and highest expected measurements. If the relationship between the actual and measured values for a quantity is consistent in a rigorous (mathematical) manner, then it may be sufficient to calibrate an instrument at only a few points.

Linearity

If the numerical values of the calibration points and the numerical values of the readings obtained with an instrument lie in a straight line when they are graphed, the instrument is said to be *linear*. Most instruments are nearly linear only over a certain range of values, and the manufacturer often specifies this range. If a reasonably linear response can be assumed for an instrument, it is necessary to calibrate it only at two points and assume that all other measurements lie on the line through these points. In actual practice, because instruments are not perfectly linear, and because measurements are seldom exactly reproducible, a *line of best fit* is often drawn to describe data points from the readings of an instrument as compared to the actual values of the calibration standards. The graphs in figure 2.1 depict various examples of lines and curves that could be present when calibrating exercise-testing equipment. The x-axis represents five standards that increase an equal amount from one measurement to the next. The y-axis presents the measure taken by the instrument that is being calibrated. Figure 2.1a depicts a positive linear relationship, which means that as one measure increases, the

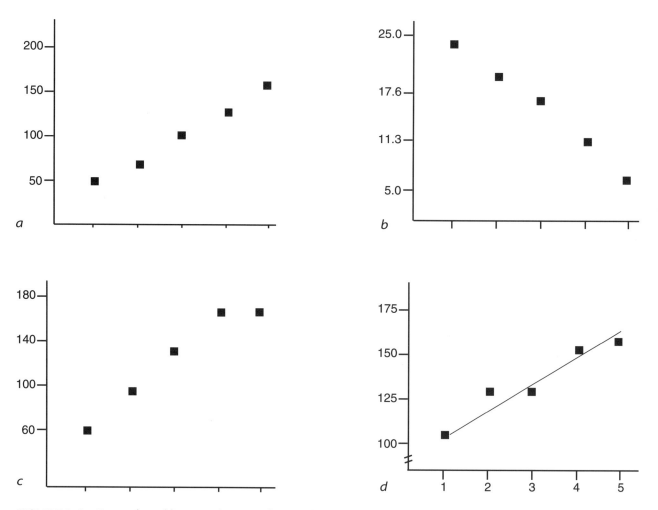

FIGURE 2.1   Examples of lines and curves that could be present when calibrating exercise-testing equipment: a positive linear relationship *(a)*, a negative relationship *(b)*, a curvilinear relationship *(c)*, and varying points whose relationship can most accurately be represented with a line of best fit *(d)*.

other measure also increases to the same degree. Figure 2.1b depicts a negative relationship, which indicates that as one variable increases, the other decreases. Figure 2.1c depicts a curvilinear relationship, which indicates that the device you are calibrating measures accurately only within a specific range (e.g., skinfold calipers often are not accurate beyond a specific range). Figure 2.1d depicts varying points whose relationship can best be represented with a line of best fit. Not every point will fit on the line. Very sensitive instruments often require the use of a line of best fit.

Procedures

1. Follow the instructions for calibration of the following equipment.
2. Complete the worksheets provided for each instrument.

Cycle Ergometer

This procedure applies to the steps for calibrating the belt resistance on a belt-braked bike (e.g., Monark, Tunturi). Note that both ends of the belt that passes around the rim of the wheels are attached to a revolving drum to which a pendulum is fixed. Thus, the device acts as a pendulum scale, measuring the difference in tractive efforts (resistance slowing down the wheel) at the two ends of the belt. The belt can be stretched with the lever that is adjusted with the handwheel. The deflection of the pendulum is read on a scale graduated in kiloponds (kp; equal to a kilogram) and Newtons (N). The braking power (kp) multiplied by the distance pedaled gives the amount of work in kilopond meters (kpm).

1. Be sure the bike is sitting on a level surface.
2. Remove the forward attachment of the belt from the pendulum.
3. Attach at least two different known calibration weights to the pendulum, and read the scale.
4. Record the reading of the measured weights displayed on the scale (figure 2.2).
5. If the scale does not read accurately, calibration will be required.
6. With a person sitting on the bike without feet touching the pedals, change the zero mark on the scale with the calibration gauge adjustor so that it coincides with the mark on the pendulum weight.

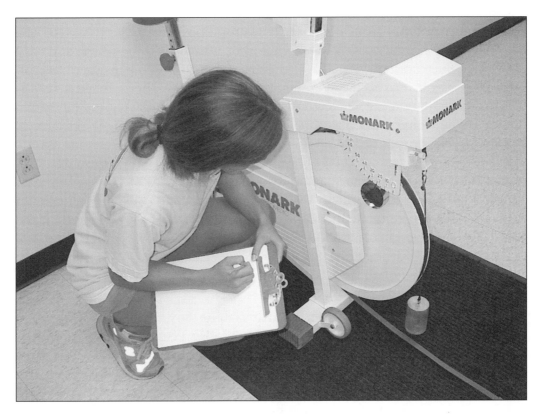

FIGURE 2.2   Cycle ergometer calibration.

7. Attach a known weight to the pendulum and read the scale. Record the reading of the measured weights displayed on the scale.

8. Check the linearity by hanging at least two different weights and recording the scale readings.

9. Graph the results of both measures by plotting the actual resistance of the known calibration weights (x-axis) against the scale readings (y-axis). The graph should represent a positive linear relationship (figure 2.1*a*, page 10).

Sphygmomanometer

A *sphygmomanometer* is a blood pressure measurement system composed of an inflatable rubber bladder, an instrument to indicate applied pressure, an inflation bulb to create pressure, and an adjustment valve to deflate the system. Of these, the cuff and the pressure-measuring instrument are the most crucial to the accuracy of the measurement (Perloff et al. 1993). To ensure accurate measurements, you must use the appropriate cuff size. When inflated the bladder should encircle at least 80% of the upper arm and not cause a bulging or displacement. If the bladder is too wide, blood pressure will be underestimated; if too narrow, pressure will be overestimated. Consequently, bladder sizes vary for children (arm girth 13-20 cm; 8 cm wide by 13 cm long), adults (arm girth 24-32 cm; 13 cm wide by 24 cm long), and large adults (arm girth 32-42 cm; 17 cm wide by 32 cm long). The pressure-measuring device can be of the mercury or aneroid type (ACSM 2000).

The mercury type is the standard. Its calibration is easily maintained. The mercury column should rise and fall smoothly, form a clear meniscus, and read zero when the bladder is deflated. If sticking occurs, clean the inside of the column according to the specific manufacturer's recommendations. If mercury falls below zero, add mercury. The mercurial sphygmomanometer should be read at the top of the mercury bubble as the level falls. The aneroid gauge uses a metal bellows assembly that expands when pressure is applied. A spring moves the attached pointer to zero when the bladder is deflated. This gauge should be calibrated once every 6 months at a variety of settings using a mercury column. A simple Y tube is used to connect the two systems together. Take readings with pressure falling to simulate the readings during an actual measurement. If the aneroid gauge is not in calibration, return it to the manufacturer for calibration, or dispose of and replace it.

Scale

A scale is a measuring instrument used to determine the gross weight of an object. The instrument can be digital, as in the case of a load cell; spring resistance, as in a Chatillon scale; or a balance beam scale (commonly found in a physician's office). Maintain the accuracy of the instruments through daily assessment and calibration. The digital scale, or load cell, usually has a self-calibration system that is found within the device or a calibration button that resets the scale to zero.

To calibrate this type of scale, either turn the device off and back on, or press the reset button. The Chatillon scale measures weight through pressure resistance on an internal spring system. This type of scale has an adjustment screw or knob that can be turned to calibrate the unweighted device display to zero. The balance beam scale, often referred to as a physician's scale, has an adjustment screw on the end of the balance beam. With the scale unweighted and the slide weights set at zero, turn the adjustment screw until the beam arm is centered, indicating that the device is zeroed. After the instruments have been calibrated, you can use a set of known weight standards to verify the calibration. The weights can be either suspended from the device or placed on the platform, depending on the instrument. When verifying the calibration, use at least two different known weights.

Discussion Questions

1. Why is calibration important?
2. Describe and give examples of sources of random error and systematic error.
3. What does lack of linearity suggest about the accuracy of a lab instrument or technique?
4. Describe what a line of best fit represents.
5. Did the instruments tested require calibration? Please explain either a yes or no answer.

Bibliography

ACSM (American College of Sports Medicine). 2000. *ACSM's Guidelines for Exercise Testing and Prescription*, 6th ed. Baltimore: Lippincott Williams & Wilkins.

Perloff, D., C. Grim, J. Flack, E.D. Frohlich, M. Hill, M. MacDonald, and B.Z. Morgenstern. 1993. Human blood pressure determination by sphygmomanometry. *Circulation* 88: 2460-2470.

Risk Factor Evaluation, Medical History, and Informed Consent

PURPOSE

This lab presents the appropriate procedures and specific content necessary for gaining the client's informed consent. This lab includes case studies in which you will be required to evaluate the client's risk factors and place him or her in the appropriate classification.

MATERIALS

1. *ACSM's Guidelines for Exercise Testing and Prescription* (6th ed.), chapters 1, 2, 3, 13
2. One copy of the Medical History Form (page 117) or the Health Screening Form (page 116)
3. One copy of the Informed Consent Form (page 120)

4. One copy of the Physician Release Form (page 121)
5. Twelve copies of the Risk Stratification Form (page 122)

Background Information

Risk stratification was developed for exercise professionals in an attempt to improve safety and reduce the risk of injury for clients before they undergo exercise testing and physical activity. Risk stratification is based on known factors that predict cardiovascular disease such as age, family history, previous and current health status, medical history, and current activity levels (Howley and Franks 2003). From this information the exercise professional can classify an individual into one of three categories. The ACSM (2000) has developed tables that allow the exercise professional to make the best decision as to the appropriate classification category for each individual client. This classification category gives guidance to the exercise professional on whether a physician should be present and what type of exercise regimen should be followed.

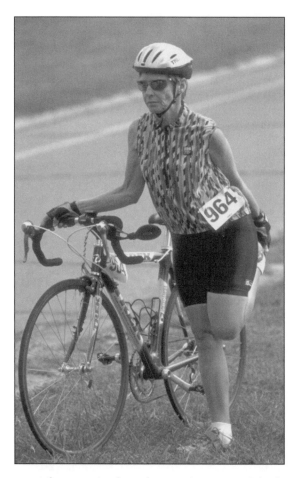

FIGURE 3.1   If you prescribe exercise based on an incorrect risk classification, you will be placing your client's health in danger.

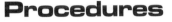

Procedures

1. The lab instructor gives a short lecture on risk-factor evaluation and informed consent.
2. The lab instructor explains the use of the following forms:
    a. Medical History Form (page 117) and Health Screening Form, which can be used if a shorter form is desired (page 116)
    b. Physician Release Form (page 121)
    c. Risk Stratification Form (page 122)
    d. Informed Consent Form (page 120)
3. The lab instructor presents case studies 1 through 12 (pages 20-29).

Assignment for Case Studies and Pretest Evaluation

Complete or answer the following for each of the 12 case studies. You will note a great deal of variation in the medical histories and case studies. Throughout your career, the information you will have available or will be able to obtain on clients will also vary widely. By dealing with the range of styles and levels of information completeness presented in these case studies, you will become more proficient at reading different types of reports and assessing the pertinent information for the purpose of risk stratification.

1. Complete a Risk Stratification Form for each case study.
2. Would you recommend a medical examination and exercise testing before the client begins moderate exercise? Vigorous exercise?
3. Would you recommend physician supervision of submaximal exercise test? Maximal exercise test?
4. What are some other areas of concern you may need to address? Does this client require referral for further health or nutritional counseling?

Before evaluating the 12 case studies, become familiar with table 3.1, *ACSM's Initial Risk Stratification* (page 17), ACSM's recommendations regarding preparticipation medical exams and exercise testing and physician supervision of exercise (table 3.2, page 17), and table 3.3, *Coronary Artery Disease Risk Factor Thresholds for Use With ACSM Risk Stratification* (page 18). Through years of clinical research and professional experience, ACSM has developed these guidelines and recommendations. The Risk Stratification table allows fitness professionals to categorize individuals according to risk factors and signs or symptoms to aid in triage and other decision-making processes. The recommendations in table 3.2 provide general guidance on the need for a medical examination and exercise testing before participation in a moderate-to-vigorous exercise program.

TABLE 3.1

ACSM's Initial Risk Stratification

Low risk	Men <45 yr of age or women <55 yr of age who are asymptomatic and meet no more than one risk factor threshold from table 3.3
Moderate risk	Older individuals (men ≥45 yr; women ≥55 yr) or those who meet the threshold for two or more risk factors from table 3.3

High risk	Individuals with
	• known cardiac, peripheral vascular, or cerebrovascular disease; chronic obstructive pulmonary disease, asthma, interstitial lung disease, or cystic fibrosis; or diabetes mellitus (types 1 and 2), thyroid disorders, or renal or liver disease, or
	• one or more of the following signs or symptoms:
	  - heart murmur;
	  - unexplained fatigue;
	  - dizziness or fainting;
	  - swelling of the ankles;
	  - fast or irregular heartbeat;
	  - unexplained shortness of breath;
	  - intermittent lameness or pain in calf muscles;
	  - breathing discomfort when not in upright position, or interrupted breathing at night; or
	  - pain or discomfort in the jaw, neck, chest, arms, or elsewhere that could be caused by lack of circulation.

Adapted, by permission, from American College of Sports Medicine, 2000, *ACSM's guidelines for exercise testing and prescription*, 6th ed. (Philadelphia, PA: Lippincott, Williams, and Wilkins), 26.

TABLE 3.2

ACSM's Recommendations

	Low risk	Moderate risk	High risk
Current (within past year) medical examination and exercise testing before participation			
Moderate exercise	Not necessary[1]	Not necessary	Recommended[2]
Vigorous exercise	Not necessary	Recommended	Recommended
Physician supervision of exercise tests			
Submaximal test	Not necessary	Not necessary	Recommended
Maximal test	Not necessary	Recommended	Recommended

[1]The designation *not necessary* reflects that a medical examination, exercise test, and physician supervision of the exercise test are not essential in the preparticipation screening but should not be viewed as inappropriate.

[2]When physician supervision of exercise testing is *recommended,* the physician should be readily available in close proximity should an emergent need develop.

Adapted, by permission, from American College of Sports Medicine, 2000, *ACSM's guidelines for exercise testing and prescription*, 6th ed. (Philadelphia, PA: Lippincott, Williams, and Wilkins), 27.

TABLE 3.3

Coronary Artery Disease Risk Factor Thresholds for Use With ACSM Risk Stratification

Risk factors	Defining criteria
Positive Family history	Myocardial infarction, coronary revascularization, or sudden death before 55 yr of age in father or other male first-degree relative (i.e., brother or son), or before 65 yr of age in mother or other female first-degree relative (i.e., sister or daughter)
Cigarette smoking	Current cigarette smoker or those who quit within the previous 6 mo
Hypertension	Systolic blood pressure of ≥140 mmHg or diastolic ≥90 mmHg, confirmed by measurements on at least 2 separate occasions, or on antihypertensive medication
Hypercholesterolemia	Total serum cholesterol of >200 mg/dL (5.2 mmol/L) or high-density lipoprotein cholesterol of <35 mg/dL (0.9 mmol/L), or on lipid-lowering medication; if low-density lipoprotein cholesterol is available, use >130 mg/dL (3.4 mmol/L) rather than total cholesterol of >200 mg/dL
Impaired fasting glucose	Fasting blood glucose of ≥110 mg/dL (6.1 mmol/L) confirmed by measurements on at least 2 separate occasions
Obesity[†]	Body mass index of ≥30 kg/m^2, or waist girth of >100 cm
Sedentary lifestyle	Persons not participating in a regular exercise program or meeting the minimal physical activity recommendations[‡] from the U.S. Surgeon General's report
Negative High serum HDL cholesterol[§]	>60 mg/dL (1.6 mmol/L)

Reprinted, by permission, from American College of Sports Medicine, 2000, *ACSM's Guidelines for exercise testing and prescription,* 6th ed. Philadelphia: Lippincott, Williams, and Wilkins, 24. Adapted from Expert Panel on Detection, Evaluation, and Treatment of High Blood Cholesterol in Adults. Summary of the second report of the National Cholesterol Education Program (NCEP) expert panel on detection, evaluation, and treatment of high blood cholesterol in adults (Adult Treatment Panel II). JAMA 1993; 269:3015-3023.

[†]Professional opinions vary regarding the most appropriate markers and thresholds for obesity; therefore, exercise professionals should use clinical judgment when evaluating this risk factor.

[‡]Accumulating 30 minutes or more of moderate physical activity on most days of the week.

[§]It is common to sum risk factors in making clinical judgments. If high-density lipoprotein (HDL) cholesterol is high, subtract one risk factor from the sum of positive risk factors because high HDL decreases CAD risk.

In studying table 3.2, it is important to note that *moderate exercise* is defined as activities that are approximately 3-6 metabolic equivalents (METs) or the equivalent of brisk walking at 3-4 mph for most healthy adults. Nevertheless, some sedentary or older persons might consider a pace of 3-4 mph to be "hard" to "very hard." Moderate exercise may alternatively be defined as an intensity well within the client's capacity, one that the client can comfortably sustain for a prolonged period (about 45 min), has a gradual initiation and progression, and is generally noncompetitive. If a person's exercise capacity is known, relative moderate exercise may be defined by the range 40-60% maximal oxygen uptake. *Vigorous exercise* is defined as activities of greater than 6 METs or, alternatively, as exercise intense enough to represent a substantial cardiorespiratory challenge. If a person's exercise capacity is known, vigorous exercise may be defined as an intensity of greater than 60% maximum oxygen uptake.

Case Studies

Case Study 1

Demography

Age: 24
Ht: 5 ft 8 in.
Sex: Female
Race: White
Wt: 109 lb

Family History

This client has no family history of cardiovascular disease.

Medical History

Present Conditions

This woman's resting heart rate (HR) is 65 bpm, and her resting blood pressure (BP) is 104/62. She has a total cholesterol of 220 mg/dl. Her high-density lipoprotein (HDL) level is 45 mg/dl and triglycerides are 120 mg/dl. She recently had a maximal oxygen consumption test that indicates her $\dot{V}O_2$max is 48 ml/kg/min. The maximal stress test indicates no known cardiovascular or electrocardiogram (ECG) abnormalities.

Past Conditions

The client has reported no past medical problems.

Behavior and Risk Factor Assessment

The client reports that she is not a smoker but she likes to have a cocktail after she leaves work. She states that she doesn't really like the bar she frequents because of the heavy secondhand smoke she has to breathe. She currently eats a diet that is rich in complex carbohydrates and lean sources of protein. Her personal trainer has her eating 4-5 meals per day. She likes to run 3-5 miles a day at least 4 days per week, and she does resistance-training exercises 5 days a week. Her job requires her to work between 50 and 60 hours per week. She sleeps an average of 6 hours each night. Her greatest concern is that she feels tired all the time.

Case Study 2

Demography

Age: 32
Ht: 5 ft 5 in.
Sex: Female
Race: White
Wt: 128 lb

Family History

Father (age 56) and mother (age 56) are both living and are very active and healthy. Two sisters (ages 30 and 28) are also both very active and healthy.

Medical History

Present Conditions

The client is presently 4 weeks pregnant and is consulting her physician to obtain approval to continue in her aerobics exercise classes at a local health facility. Examinations revealed the following information about this woman:

Resting HR: 76   Resting BP: 108/72

Total cholesterol: 178 mg/dl   HDL cholesterol: 72 mg/dl

Triglycerides: 76 mg/dl   Body fat: 22%

Past Conditions

This client has been well throughout her life. She did have one full-term pregnancy and delivered a healthy baby 3 yr ago. During her first pregnancy she was continuously active until her eighth month, at which time her physician told her to "slow down." She loves aerobics and wants to stay in shape. Her MET level is currently 13.

Behavior and Risk-Factor Assessment

This client has been participating in aerobics for 7 yr on a regular basis. She has never had shinsplints or other orthopedic problems. She did experience some light-headedness and lower back pain during her first pregnancy, but she intends, during this pregnancy, to follow guidelines more carefully regarding appropriate exercises. She does not smoke or drink alcoholic beverages. She tries to nap 30 min during the afternoon and also takes walks whenever she can. She has recently started experiencing some problems with morning sickness.

Physical Exam

A recent physical examination to determine her present health status and to follow her progress during pregnancy showed that she had gained 5 lb during the past month. She has normal resting BP and HR readings. The doctor has approved continuation in her aerobics program providing she follows safety guidelines.

Case Study 3

Demography

Age: 31
Ht: 6 ft
Sex: Male
Race: Black
Wt: 155 lb

Family History

Both parents are still alive and have had no known cardiovascular disease. An older brother died from a massive myocardial infarction (MI) at the age of 44.

Medical History

Present Conditions

The blood lipid profile reveals a total cholesterol of 145 mg/dl, HDL of 45 mg/dl, triglycerides of 60 mg/dl, and blood glucose of 80 mg/dl. Resting BP is measured at 124/78. The resting ECG reveals a resting HR of 42 bpm with probable left ventricular hypertrophy. The client's current body fat level is 10.5%. During the past 3 yr, the client has had recurrent stress fractures in both tibias and was recently diagnosed with anterior compartmental syndrome in both shins.

Past Conditions

The client has had no identified cardiovascular-related problems in the past. He has recurrent stress fractures of the tibias.

Behavior and Risk Factor Assessment

This man has never smoked, and he has been a competitive middle-distance runner since the age of 15. He recently had a maximal oxygen consumption test performed and achieved a 60 ml/kg/min relative $\dot{V}O_2$max. His diet consists primarily of complex carbohydrates and low-fat protein sources such as chicken and fish. He sleeps approximately 7 hours each night.

As the regional sales representative for a sporting goods manufacturer, this client experiences a great deal of pressure to maintain sales quotas. To relieve the stress of his position, he runs 10-15 miles a day.

Case Study 4

Demography

Age: 57
Ht: 5 ft 9 in.
Sex: Male
Race: White
Wt: 165 lb

Family History

This client's father died of a heart attack at the age of 42. His mother died of spinal meningitis at the age of 55. He has two siblings, a brother who is 50 yr old and a sister who is 55.

Medical History

Present Conditions

This man has been in apparently good health all his life and has had periodic ECGs performed at his place of employment. At this time the client denies any cardiorespiratory complaints—specifically, chest pain, chest pressure, or discomfort—but occasionally he has shortness of breath and cramps in his lower legs. He currently has no restrictions placed on him but has a functioning MET level of 5.

The client is on no medication and follows a low-cholesterol diet. His present lipids indicate cholesterol of 232 mg and triglycerides of 144 mg. HDL are 42 mg, and low-density lipoproteins (LDL) are 190 mg. He arrives for the test in a fasting state.

Past Conditions

At the age of 33 the subject underwent an appendectomy, which kept him in the hospital for 11.5 mos.

Behavior and Risk-Factor Assessment

The client reports he has been a cigarette smoker since the age of 14, currently smoking approximately 35-40 cigarettes a day plus cigars. His physician has advised him to stop smoking, but he indicates that smoking reduces his daily stress. He drinks liquor, wine, and beer, consuming approximately 5-6 glasses of rye or wine a day and 15-18 glasses of beer a week. His meal patterns consist of large business lunches almost daily, and a sandwich or soup for dinner. He sleeps approximately 5 hours a night, which is often disrupted because he frequently works 12-14 hours a day.

As a sales executive covering a region that stretches from the entire East Coast out to the Midwest, this client follows tight schedules and is constantly under a great deal of pressure. He travels 75% of the time, which consists of both driving and flying long distances.

Case Study 5

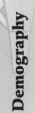

Demography

Age: 40
Ht: 6 ft 4 in.
Sex: Male
Race: White
Wt: 225 lb

Family History

This man's father had a heart attack at age 52 and underwent a five-vessel coronary bypass graft surgery at the age of 60. His mother died of a heart attack at the age of 39. He has two sisters, one age 34 and one age 30, who are both healthy.

Medical History

Present Conditions

This client is in generally good health. He has no restrictions placed on him at this time. This client eats no red meat or fried foods and uses no caffeine products. His present cholesterol level is 205 mg/dl and triglycerides are 38 mg/dl.

Past Conditions

In the past the client has had several bouts of gastritis. He had reconstructive surgery performed on his right knee at the age of 24 and still experiences an occasional recurrence of pain. At age 25 he was diagnosed as hypertensive. At that time his BP at rest was 148/92 and during stressful situations could increase to as high as 170/105. At age 25 he began taking a diuretic to maintain his BP at 120/80. At age 30 his medication was changed to a beta-blocker. His BP while on this medication has stabilized at 115/60.

Behavior and Risk Factor Assessment

This man has never smoked. He drinks 3-6 cans of beer on the weekend but never drinks any alcoholic beverages during the week. He eats a small breakfast, no lunch, and a moderate-size dinner of primarily vegetables, chicken, or fish. He does, however, salt his food heavily. He sleeps 6-7 hours a night. This client averages 12 hours a day at his office, where he is responsible for a large outpatient hospital department.

With regard to exercise, this client jogs 3 miles a day, 5 days a week, before work. He also skips rope for 20 min, 3 days a week, at noon. He presently has a body composition of 14.6% body fat. He has lost approximately 40 lb in the last 2 yr. He has a functional MET level of 12.

Physical Exam

The physical exam reveals a highly fit white male with BP of 116/60 and pulse 48 and regular. ECG is normal. The orthopedic exam reveals good flexibility and minor limitations on the right knee. The extremities show good pulses.

Case Study 6

Demography

Age: 42
Ht: 5 ft 4 in.
Sex: Female
Race: Black
Wt: 124 lb

Family History

This client's father is living (age 67) and apparently healthy, except for a recent diagnosis of moderate hypertension that is being treated with appropriate medications, altered diet, and moderate exercise. Her mother died 2 yr ago, at age 59, from breast cancer. The client has twin sisters, age 47, who are both very active and healthy.

Medical History

Present Conditions

Recently, the client has noticed considerable lack of energy and loss of incentive to exercise. Her friend has encouraged her to join a local aerobics program designed for middle-aged adults. She recently underwent an examination by her physician to determine the suitability of an exercise program for her. She has a maximal MET level of 6. Healthy screening tests indicate the following information:

Resting BP: 132/88	Resting HR: 102
Triglycerides: 185 mg/dl	HDL cholesterol: 40 mg/dl
Cholesterol ratio: 4:1	Body fat: 30%

Past Conditions

This client apparently has never been hospitalized for any reason. She has indicated that she had the typical childhood illnesses when she was young. Her biggest complaint over the years is that she experiences regular migraine headaches. She also has been taking allergy shots for environmental allergies.

Behavior and Risk-Factor Assessment

This client notes that she is a sporadic exerciser who does not seem to have the motivation to work hard during exercise. She smokes occasionally when out to dinner or at a social gathering—approximately 12-15 cigarettes a month. She drinks a glass of wine with lunch every day and has an additional glass or two of wine with dinner on the weekends. She works 70-75 hours a week, with only Sundays off to "rest." She usually spends her day off doing housework and grocery shopping. Her typical daily intake of nutrients includes mostly protein (in the form of cheese, eggs, or steak) and simple carbohydrates (such as fruit, cookies, and cake). She is disgusted with her lifestyle and desires to start feeling healthier.

Physical Exam

A postural assessment reveals that she stands with hyperextended knees and one shoulder visibly elevated higher than the other.

Case Study 7

Demography

Age: 61
Ht: 5 ft 9 in.
Sex: Male
Race: Asian American
Wt: 170 lb

Family History

This client's father died 7 yr ago (at age 81), and his mother is still living at age 86. The father died of massive coronary arrest; the mother's only complaint is mildly elevated BP, which she is treating with dietary modification. The client's only sibling is a younger brother, age 58, who is apparently healthy and quite physically active.

Medical History

Present Conditions

This apparently healthy gentleman has decided to join the local YMCA's new program, "Gentle Aerobics for Seniors." The YMCA instructor requires anyone wishing to join the program to undergo a complete physical checkup, including a monitored treadmill or cycle ergometer exercise stress test. The preliminary test administered prior to exercise stress testing revealed the following information:

Resting HR: 88   Resting BP: 140/86
Total cholesterol: 220 mg/dl   HDL cholesterol: 90 mg/dl
Triglycerides: 160 mg/dl   Fasting blood glucose: 100 mg/dl

Past Conditions

This client never had any broken bones but has had repeated problems with stiffness and soreness in the right wrist and the fingers on both hands.

Behavior and Risk Factor Assessment

The client has never smoked and drinks one to two highballs a week. He tries to watch his diet fairly carefully. He walks 1 mile (at a 15-min-mile pace) twice daily at least four times a week. When he was in college, he competed as a nationally ranked swimmer.

Physical Exam

This man has normal resting and exercise stress test ECGs. His muscles lack normal tone, and his abdominal area appears excessively large. Other than these findings, the client is apparently healthy. The stress test results indicate a maximal MET level of 8.

Case Study 8

Age: 55
Ht: 6 ft 2 in.
Sex: Male
Race: White
Wt: 230 lb

Family History

This man's father died from heart disease at age 61. His mother is still alive at the age of 75. He has no siblings.

Medical History

Present Conditions

This client has no personal history of coronary heart disease. His blood lipid profile indicates a total cholesterol value of 243 mg/dl, HDL of 31 mg/dl, triglycerides of 123 mg/dl, and blood glucose of 150 mg/dl. Three years ago, the subject's resting BP was measured at 155/98; his physician put him on hydrodiuril, and today his resting BP is 128/84. A resting ECG reveals several premature ventricular beats, approximately 30 per minute. He reports no history of chest pain but has noticed some shortness of breath lately when climbing stairs.

Behavior and Risk Factor Assessment

This man used to smoke but quit 2 yr ago. He also likes to drink a glass of wine with dinner each night. He does not perform regular aerobic exercise but performs strenuous isometric exercises 3 days a week. His current body fat level has been measured at 27%. He recently had a maximal $\dot{V}O_2$ test performed, and the results indicate his maximal MET level is 6.

Case Study 9

Age: 36
Ht: 4 ft 7 in.
Sex: Female
Race: Asian American
Wt: 164 lb

Family History

This client's father and mother are alive at the age of 75 and 74, respectively. She has no brothers or sisters.

Medical History

Present Conditions

This woman recently had a blood lipid profile that revealed a total cholesterol of 210 mg/dl, HDL cholesterol of 45 mg/dl, triglycerides of 200 mg/dl, and blood glucose of 105 mg/dl. She reports occasional palpitations in her chest during the morning, but she has no chest pain or history of heart problems. A recent graded stress test was negative for any cardiac abnormalities. The stress test also measured her $\dot{V}O_2$max at 21 ml/kg/min.

Past Conditions

The client reports a history of anorexia and bulimia in the past but states she has conquered her problem through therapy and no longer restricts her caloric intake.

Behavior and Risk Factor Assessment

This client works as a stockbroker in a large city. She drinks four cups of coffee each morning. Breakfast usually consists of a doughnut or a meal from a fast-food restaurant. She typically eats at a fast-food restaurant for lunch, since she usually takes only 30 min or less for her lunch break. She compensates for the short lunches by eating a honey bun during her coffee break. Dinner usually consists of soup and a sandwich. She consumes approximately 15 beers a week. She is sedentary but wishes to begin an exercise program to look and feel better. She has never smoked, but some of the workers in her office are moderate smokers.

Case Study 10

Demography

Age: 26
Ht: 5 ft 10 in.
Sex: Male
Race: Hispanic
Wt: 230 lb

Family History

The client has no known relatives because he was adopted at birth. He was raised by his adoptive parents, both of whom died in an auto accident before they were 45 yr of age.

Medical History

Present Conditions

The client's resting BP and HR are 160/80 and 70, respectively. His absolute $\dot{V}O_2$ is 2.3 L/min. Total cholesterol is 242 mg/dl, HDL value is 45, triglycerides are 225 mg/dl, and blood glucose is 88 mg/dl.

Past Conditions

This man had corrective surgery 5 months ago on the sinus cavity to relieve chronic snoring.

Behavior and Risk Factor Assessment

The client smokes approximately 1 pack of cigarettes a week and does not consider this a problem because "it's only a few cigarettes per day." He is considering trying the "Beverly Hills diet," which consists of nothing but fruit, because he heard that many celebrities lost weight following this regimen. He also reports that he tries to stay away from starchy carbohydrate foods because they are high in calories. Influenced by an advertisement he saw in a "muscle" magazine, he takes several amino acid supplement capsules each day in the hopes that doing so will lead to increased muscle mass. He does no strength training or aerobic activity. His body fat level is 30%. He plans on wearing a rubber suit in the summer in an attempt to shed his excess weight and body fat.

Case Study 11

Family History

This client's father died at age 35 from an MI. His mother is still alive at age 80 with no cardiovascular problems. He has an older brother who is 55 and a younger sister who is 35. Neither has reported any cardiovascular problems.

Medical History

Present Conditions
The client has a resting HR of 78 bpm. His resting BP is 146/98. A fasting blood lipid profile reveals total cholesterol of 238 mg/dl, HDL cholesterol of 13 mg/dl, triglycerides of 214 mg/dl, and a blood glucose value of 256 mg/dl.

Past Conditions
This client has not had a physical exam in 5 yr. The exam 5 yr ago revealed multiple premature ventricular contractions. He opted not to seek further medical attention. At the time of the exam the client performed at a maximum MET level of 3.5.

Behavior and Risk Factor Assessment

The client reports being a heavy chain smoker of at least 2 packs of cigarettes a day. He also likes to drink at least 6 cups of coffee every morning before going to his job at a bakery. He states he likes the job because "the fringe benefit is free pastries any time." He eats three times a day, mostly fast food in between his pastry snacks. A body fat analysis done at a company health fair indicated his body fat is approximately 35%.

Case Study 12

Family History

This client's father died of a massive heart attack at the age of 40. His mother died of cancer at age 48. His 32-year-old brother recently underwent quadruple bypass surgery for blocked coronary arteries.

Medical History

Present History
This man's blood cholesterol measures 344 mg/dl, with an HDL value of 16 mg/dl. Triglycerides are 244 mg/dl, and blood glucose level

is 159 mg/dl. Liver enzymes in the blood are greatly elevated, as are blood uric and creatinine levels. His resting BP is 170/98 and resting HR is 101 bpm.

Past Conditions

This client has experienced no previous problems.

Behavior and Risk Factor Assessment

The client is an avid powerlifter who recently won a national championship in his weight division and wants to go on to compete in the world championships. In an attempt to increase his strength, he has begun taking "black-market steroids" (prescription drugs purchased illegally without a prescription) without medical supervision. He has noticed a marked increase in his strength when lifting weights but is bothered by the frequent nosebleeds he gets while training. His diet consists primarily of hamburgers, french fries, and milk shakes. He does no aerobic training. He drinks alcohol occasionally but states, "I only drink whiskey and Diet Coke, so that isn't so bad."

Discussion Questions

Respond to and discuss the following questions:

1. To give valid consent to a procedure, what characteristics must a client maintain?
2. What are the seven components of a valid informed consent procedure and form?
3. What should be included in a medical history evaluation?
4. What are the components of the physical exam and the laboratory tests?

Bibliography

ACSM (American College of Sports Medicine). 2000. *ACSM's Guidelines for Exercise Testing and Prescription*, 6th ed. Baltimore: Lippincott, Williams & Wilkins.

Howley, E.T., and B.D. Franks. 2003. *Health Fitness Instructors Handbook*, 4th ed. Champaign, IL: Human Kinetics.

PART II

Techniques in Exercise Testing

PART II comprises six labs that focus on the techniques used to assess the components of health-related fitness (cardiorespiratory function, muscular strength and endurance, flexibility, and body composition), including information on ECG placement and operating ECG equipment. The application procedures in these labs include step-by-step instructions, diagrams depicting appropriate techniques, and charts that present norms for making comparisons by age and gender. Forms for recording data are in appendix A. Because many of these forms will be used more than once during the course, make photocopies before using them.

Introduction to Health Fitness Assessment Techniques

PURPOSE

This lab introduces students to the specific measurement techniques for assessing HR, BP, skinfolds, and circumferences.

MATERIALS

1. Skinfold calipers
2. Gulick tape
3. Stopwatch
4. Stethoscope
5. Sphygmomanometer
6. Cycle ergometer
7. One copy of the Skinfold and Circumference Data Collection Worksheet (page 136)
8. One copy of the Heart Rate and Blood Pressure Data Collection Worksheet (page 137)

Background Information

Understanding and becoming familiar with equipment and devices used to collect data for evaluation is very important. Through repeated practice with the devices and guidance from a qualified instructor, an exercise professional develops the skills necessary to accurately test and measure the specific variables, and eventually becomes successful and proficient in the area of exercise testing.

Skinfold and Circumference

Body fat levels and fat distribution are recognized as valid predictors of health risks associated with obesity (ACSM 2000). The diseases associated with high

TABLE 4.1

Standardized Description of Sites for Body Composition Measurements

Skinfold sites	
Abdominal	A vertical fold taken at a distance of 2 cm to the right side of the umbilicus
Biceps	A vertical fold taken on the anterior aspect of the arm over the belly of the biceps muscle, 1 cm above the level used to mark the triceps
Chest/pectoral	A diagonal fold taken one-half the distance between the anterior axillary line and the nipple in men, and one-third of the distance between the anterior axillary line and the nipple in women
Medial calf	A vertical fold at a level of the maximum circumference of the calf on the midline of its medial border
Midaxillary	A vertical fold taken on the midaxillary line at the level of the xiphoid process of the sternum
Subscapular	An angular fold taken at a 45-degree angle 1–2 cm below the inferior angle of the scapula
Supraillium	An oblique (diagonal) fold taken in the anterior axillary line superior to the iliac crest
Thigh	A vertical fold taken on the anterior midline of the thigh, midway between the proximal border of the patella and the inguinal crease (hip)
Triceps	A vertical fold taken on the posterior midline of the upper arm, halfway between the acromion and olecranon processes, with the arm held freely down the side of the body
Circumferential measuring sites	
Waist	With the subject's abdomen relaxed, a horizontal measure is taken at the narrowest part of the torso between the xiphoid process and the umbilicus.
Hip	With the subject standing erect and naturally, a horizontal measure is taken at the maximum circumference of the hips or buttocks region (whichever is larger) above the gluteal fold.

Adapted, by permission, from American College of Sports Medicine, 2000, *ACSM's guidelines for exercise testing and prescription*, 6th ed. (Philadelphia, PA: Lippincott, Williams, and Wilkins), 65.

levels of body fat include hypertension, coronary artery disease, type 2 diabetes, hyperlipidemia, and certain types of cancers (ACSM 1998; U.S. Department of Health and Human Services 1996).

Skinfold and circumference procedures provide an inexpensive method for identifying obesity risk. Table 4.1 describes the sites to use for both skinfold and circumferential measurements. The ACSM outlines specific procedures for each method (ACSM 1995):

SKINFOLD PROCEDURES

1. Take measurements on the right side of the body.
2. Place the calipers 1 cm away from the thumb and finger, perpendicular to the skinfold and halfway between the crest and the base of the fold (figure 4.1).
3. Maintain the pinch while reading the calipers.
4. Wait 1-2 seconds (and not longer) before reading calipers.
5. Take duplicate measurements at each site.
6. Retest if the measurements do not fall within 1-2 mm.
7. Rotate through the measurement sites, or allow time for the skin to regain its normal texture and thickness.
8. Record the measurements on data sheets.

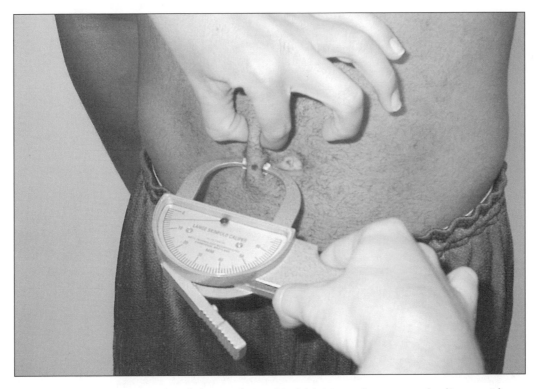

FIGURE 4.1 Measuring the abdominal site skinfold. Note placement of calipers with respect to fingers of left hand.

CIRCUMFERENTIAL TECHNIQUE

1. Pull Gulick tape to proper tension (so it is snug) without pinching the skin. Check that the tape is neither indenting the skin nor loose enough to leave gaps between the tape and skin (figure 4.2).
2. Take duplicate measurements at each site.
3. Retest if the measurements do not fall within 1 cm.
4. Record the measurements on data sheets.

When assessing body composition using either method, accuracy of technique is extremely important. To improve tester accuracy, the ACSM recommends training with a skilled technician, routinely practicing the techniques, attending workshops, and regularly demonstrating reliability (ACSM 2000, ACSM 1995).

Heart Rate

HR and work intensity are linearly related—that is, one increases proportionately with the other. By measuring HR, we can determine how hard the body is working and how it is responding to exercise. HR is a physiological parameter that is easy to monitor.

HR can be monitored by palpating a superficial artery, a procedure that is universally known as taking the pulse. During exercise, the most common site for

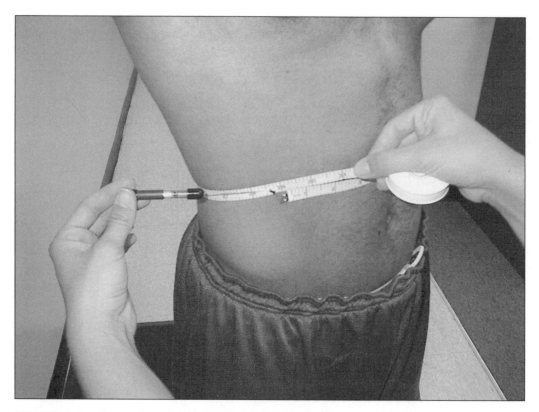

FIGURE 4.2   Circumferential measurement at the waist.

monitoring HR is the radial artery, which descends on the lateral (thumb) side of the forearm to become quite superficial at the distal end of the radius. Taking the pulse at this end consists of compressing the artery against the anterior surface of the distal end of the radius. You can also find a pulse in the temporal artery, brachial artery, femoral artery, popliteal artery, posterior tibial artery, and dorsalis pedis artery.

The common carotid arteries on both sides of the neck have anatomic landmarks that are similar to each other. The common carotid pulse in the neck is bounded by the body of the mandible (lower jaw), the sternocleidomastoid muscle, and the larynx (i.e., Adam's apple). Palpate the carotid arterial pulses by gently compressing inward and backward along the anterior border of the sternocleidomastoid muscle at the level of the thyroid cartilage.

Palpate the carotid pulses singly (one carotid artery at a time) by placing the first two fingers (not the thumb) lightly on the artery. Reports have shown that palpitation of the carotid artery after exercise has ended may produce bradycardia in some people. In addition, this method is inappropriate for participants who have various forms of vascular disease that affects the sensitivity of the carotid sinus.

Blood Pressure

BP allows us to determine how the cardiovascular system (heart and vascular system) is responding to exercise. By monitoring BP, we are able to determine whether the cardiovascular system is adapting properly to the exercise or is posing undue stress on the body. BP is an important indicator of cardiorespiratory function at rest, during physical work, and during emotional stress. Monitoring HR and BP is the easiest and quickest method of assessing an individual's health and exercise status.

When measuring BP, wrap the blood pressure cuff snugly around the person's upper arm, locating the center of the cuff bladder over the brachial artery and the bottom of the cuff 1 in. above the antecubital fossa (fold in the arm). Tighten the valve on the bulb and begin to inflate. Place the head of the stethoscope on the brachial artery (located between the midline and the medial portion of the antecubital space). Inflate the cuff to the point at which the pulse disappears, then add an additional 20-30 mmHg (200 mmHg). The 200 mmHg will be read from the mercury column or the anaeroid scale. This represents the amount of pressure required to raise a column of mercury 200 mm. Begin deflating immediately at a rate of 2-3 mmHg per second. Record the first sound heard as the systolic BP (Korotkoff phase I), or the pressure exerted against the walls of the arteries during heart muscle contraction. The disappearance of sound (Korotkoff phase V) is considered the diastolic BP, or the pressure exerted against the artery walls during the relaxation phase of the contraction. A normal BP reading is 120/80 mmHg, with 120 reflecting the systolic pressure and 80 the diastolic pressure. As you deflate the cuff by releasing the valve, watch the meter to match the sound changes with the numbers on the gauge. If you have no idea what the normal range is for the person you are testing, it is appropriate to ask. This information will decrease the risk of overinflation that may be uncomfortable.

Procedures

1. In groups of 3 to 5, practice taking skinfolds and circumferences on each other. Record your own skinfolds and circumferences on the Skinfolds and Circumference Data Collection Worksheet (page 136).

2. Follow the standard skinfold and circumferential measurement techniques outlined in this lab.

3. In the same groups of 3-5, practice taking HR and BP on each other. Record your own resting HR and BP on the Heart Rate and Blood Pressure Data-Collection Worksheet (page 137).

4. After obtaining resting data, have one person from each group exercise on a cycle ergometer for 12 min (four 3-min stages). The cycler will maintain a 50-rpm pedaling rate for the duration of the exercise. After 2-3 min of unloaded warm-up, increase the resistance to 0.5 kg during the first stage. Increase each subsequent stage by 0.5 kg (e.g., 0.5 to 1.0 kg, to 1.5 kg, etc.).

5. Monitor HR and BP during the 12 min of exercise and 3 min of recovery (reduce resistance to 0.5 kg). Take exercise HR at min 2 and 3 of each stage with BP taken at the midpoint of each workload (i.e., begin HR measurement at 1:45, 2:45, 4:45, 5:45, etc., and BP at 2:00, 5:00, etc.).

6. The timer should announce the time for the assessment of the respective parameters. Be sure to record the information on the data sheet. Remember to convert the 15-sec HR to beats per minute (bpm).

Discussion Questions

1. Describe potential sources of error in the process of taking skinfolds and circumferences.
2. The thumb should not be used for HR palpitation. Why?
3. Which HR determination method is closest to a full 60-sec count?
4. What factors can cause changes in resting BP?
5. What information do HR and BP tell us during an exercise test?

Bibliography

ACSM (American College of Sports Medicine). 1995. *ACSM's Guidelines for Exercise Testing and Prescription*, 5th ed. Baltimore: Williams & Wilkins.

ACSM (American College of Sports Medicine). 1998. *ACSM's Resource Manual for Guidelines for Exercise Testing and Prescription,* 3rd ed. Baltimore: Lippincott Williams & Wilkins.

ACSM (American College of Sports Medicine). 2000. *ACSM's Guidelines for Exercise Testing and Prescription,* 6th ed. Baltimore: Lippincott Williams & Wilkins.

U.S. Department of Health and Human Services. 1996. *Physical Activity and Health: A Report of the Surgeon General.* Washington, DC: International Medical Publishing.

Submaximal Exercise Test Protocols

PURPOSE

This lab presents two types of submaximal exercise test protocols (the Åstrand-Ryhming test and the YMCA Submaximal Cycle Ergometer Protocol) used to determine cardiovascular fitness levels, and emphasizes practice of these protocols.

MATERIALS

1. Cycle ergometer or treadmill
2. Sphygmomanometer
3. Stethoscope
4. Stopwatch
5. RPE scale
6. One copy of the Åstrand-Ryhming Data Collection Worksheet (page 138)
7. Copy of the YMCA Data Collection Worksheet (page 139)
8. Copy of the YMCA $\dot{V}O_2$max Estimation Graph (page 140)
9. ECG (if available)

Background Information

The single most scientifically accepted indicator of cardiovascular fitness is the body's ability to take in and utilize oxygen. The measurement of this ability is known as maximal oxygen consumption, or $\dot{V}O_2$max. The most widely accepted indicator for the prediction of cardiovascular fitness, however, is HR.

Maximal oxygen consumption may be defined as the maximal rate at which the body can take up, distribute, and use oxygen in the performance of large-muscle-mass exercise. For muscular work lasting more than 6 min at rates for which anaerobic sources of energy are not exceeded, there exists a highest level of work at which the body reaches its maximum capacity to supply oxygen. Levels of $\dot{V}O_2$max are observed after the participant's workload is increased progressively until it exceeds the capacity of the oxygen uptake and requires anaerobic sources of power in the final spurt. When oxygen uptake can no longer increase despite the fact that work can continue at higher levels for a short time because of anaerobic power sources, the participant has reached a plateau for maximal oxygen uptake (aerobic capacity). Every person has a measurable upper limit of oxygen uptake, which correlates with his or her ability to do aerobic work.

Factors Affecting $\dot{V}O_2$max

A person's $\dot{V}O_2$max level depends on body build and composition and is also affected by the following factors:

1. **Gender.** Comparatively, the typical female will have a lower $\dot{V}O_2$max than the normal male.
2. **Age.** The maximal oxygen uptake of a 75-year-old person is only half that of a 17-year-old person of the same sex. Recent literature suggests that improvement can be seen in prepubescent children.
3. **Size.** A person's maximal oxygen uptake is directly proportional to height and body surface area.
4. **Weight.** Maximal oxygen uptake is proportional to a person's weight.
5. **Lean body mass.** $\dot{V}O_2$max correlates 0.63 with body weight, 0.85 with fat-free body weight, and 0.91 with active muscle tissue.
6. **Bed rest.** Enforced bed rest of 3 weeks reduces maximal oxygen uptake by approximately 17%.
7. **Altitude.** At an altitude of 4,000 m, $\dot{V}O_2$max is reduced by approximately 26%. The reduction increases as altitude increases.
8. **Geography.** $\dot{V}O_2$max is reduced for residents of temperate or tropical areas as compared with those living in circumpolar regions.

Maximal oxygen uptake is not affected by the following:

1. Ingestion of a small meal (up to about 750 kcal)
2. Exposure to heat stress up to 90°F
3. Whether the participant warms up before exercise (duration of warm-up exercise can vary)

4. Speed of exercise (rate of work can be slow, moderate, or fast)
5. Repetition (retests at intervals of 20-30 min show similar results)

Maximal oxygen uptake can increase with physical conditioning or decrease with inactivity. The limiting factors may be one or both of the following:

1. The capacity of the respiratory and circulatory systems to take up and transport oxygen, a process that is dependent on alveolar ventilation, diffusing capacity of the lungs, and capacity of the blood flow for transporting oxygen from the lungs to the capillaries
2. The capacity of the working muscles to receive and use oxygen

Measuring $\dot{V}O_2$max

A maximal oxygen consumption test requires that the participant exert maximal effort in performing physical work, generally on a treadmill or bike, to exhaustion. The test begins with a relatively light workload and progresses, with increases every 2-3 min, to a workload that the participant can no longer sustain. This requires great effort by the participant. To ensure accuracy, the tester evaluates criteria to ensure that the participant has achieved a maximal level of oxygen consumption. The four most relevant criteria are

1. the plateau of oxygen consumption,
2. the attainment of respiratory exchange ratios of 1:1 or higher,
3. the attainment of age-predicted HR, and
4. the exhaustion of the participant.

Use of Spirometry in Assessing Maximal Oxygen Consumption

Maximal oxygen uptake can be measured by *open-circuit spirometry* or can be predicted from the peak exercise time or power output achieved during a standard maximal exercise test protocol (i.e., Bruce protocol). It can also be predicted from submaximal exercise tests.

The open-circuit spirometry method of measuring oxygen consumption is the most accurate means currently available for determining a person's aerobic capacity during exercise. The participant inhales ambient air composed of 20.93% oxygen, 0.03-0.04% carbon dioxide, and 79.04% nitrogen during exercise. Because the body uses the oxygen, the exhaled gases will contain less oxygen and more carbon dioxide than the inhaled air. The equipment for open-circuit spirometry is expensive and specialized and is not generally available to health and fitness specialists; therefore it will not be discussed further in this lab.

Submaximal Exercise Tests for Estimating Maximal Oxygen Consumption

A $\dot{V}O_2$max test is not practical for a large population, nor is it always safe for all participants. With this in mind, exercise technicians have developed a submaximal test that should accurately estimate a person's maximal $\dot{V}O_2$. These submaximal tests use HR responses to incremental workloads to predict percentages of $\dot{V}O_2$max. As workload increases, HR increases proportionately (positive linear relationship). Once you have established a participant's HR responses to a series of submaximal loads, you can use the slope of the line created by the HR responses to those workloads and extrapolate to the participant's age-predicted maximal HR to a prediction of $\dot{V}O_2$max. This prediction is an estimate of $\dot{V}O_2$max. The underlying basis of submaximal tests involving HR, $\dot{V}O_2$, and workload are shown in figure 5.1.

The Åstrand-Ryhming test and the YMCA Submaximal Cycle Ergometer Protocol are procedures that fitness professionals commonly use to predict $\dot{V}O_2$max.

Rating of Perceived Exertion

Another means of determining whether a participant has reached maximal oxygen uptake is through the use of a scale known as the rating of perceived exertion (RPE; see figure 5.2). This scale serves as a subjective measure of the participant's sense of effort. Someone who is performing maximal work will report maximal effort; thus this scale provides further support for the accuracy of a maximal effort test. In addition, fitness professionals can use RPE to prescribe exercise intensity.

Because maximal HR varies greatly among participants during exercise, it is helpful to be able to evaluate RPE to assess whether a test is truly maximal and when a participant is approaching maximum exercise. RPE from the category scale correlates closely with several exercise variables, including percentage

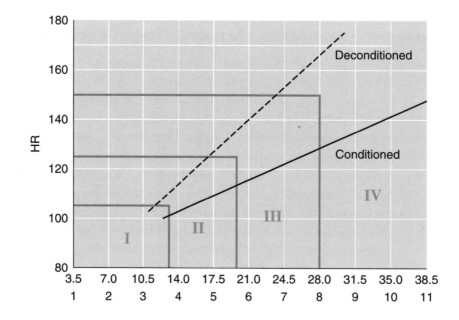

FIGURE 5.1   The linear relationship between HR and workload increases.
By measuring HR at each stage of a submaximal exercise test, you can predict a person's $\dot{V}O_2$ max by extrapolating the maximal workload to the age-predicted maximal HR.
Reprinted, by permission, from F. Cerny and H. Burton, 2001, *Exercise physiology for health care professionals* (Champaign, IL: Human Kinetics), 302.

Category Scale

6

7   Very, very light

8

9   Very light

10

11   Fairly light

12

13   Somewhat hard

14

15   Hard

16

17   Very hard

18

19   Very, very hard

20

© Borg RPE Scale
Gunnar Borg, 1970, 1985, 1994, 1998

FIGURE 5.2   Rating of perceived exertion (RPE) scale.
Reprinted, by permission, from G. Borg, 1998, *Borg's perceived exertion and pain scales* (Champaign, IL: Human Kinetics), p. 47.

of $\dot{V}O_2$peak ($\dot{V}O_2$peak is used to refer to the highest $\dot{V}O_2$ achieved during a "max" test. Often this term describes $\dot{V}O_2$ when the criterion for $\dot{V}O_2$max is not met), percentage of heart rate reserve (HRR), minute ventilation, and blood lactate levels.

During most exercise testing, the RPE scale is an accurate gauge of impeding fatigue. Clinical experience indicates, however, that 5-10% of test participants unfamiliar with the scale tend to underestimate or suppress RPE below expected levels during the early and middle stages of testing. For this reason, it is important that the participant you are testing has a clear understanding of the RPE scale and how to gauge effort. To communicate this thoroughly, first make sure that you understand the RPE scale. Then, before beginning the test, state to the subject, "While you are participating in exercise, it is quite common to have a sense of how hard you are working. I would like you to consider the total amount of exertion you feel, taking into account all sensations of physical stress, effort, and fatigue in your whole body."

Procedures

1. Determine the estimated relative and absolute $\dot{V}O_2$max from each test.
2. Before beginning the procedures, review general indications for stopping an exercise test (page 80) and absolute and relative indications for terminating

exercise testing (page 104) in *ACSM's Guidelines for Exercise Testing and Prescription, Sixth Edition*.

Following are the steps in administering three different submaximal cycle ergometer tests.

Åstrand-Ryhming Test

1. Select a participant in your group to be the test subject.
2. Adjust the seat height on the cycle ergometer. The participant should sit upright and when the foot is at the bottom of the pedaling stroke, that leg should be slightly bent at the knee, 5°.
3. Record the participant's weight and age.
4. Have the participant warm up for 2-3 min by pedaling at 50 rpm with no resistance.
5. This is a single-stage test lasting for 6 min. Instruct the participant to continue pedaling, and immediately set the resistance according to the following scale.

   Unconditioned participant

Male	300 kg/m/min (1 kp = 50 Watts) or 600 kg/m/min (2 kp = 100 Watts)
Female	300 kg/m/min (1 kp = 50 Watts) or 450 kg/m/min (1.5 kp = 75 Watts)

   Conditioned participant

Male	600 kg/m/min (2 kp = 100 Watts) or 900 kg/m/min (3 kp = 150 Watts)
Female	450 kg/m/min (1.5 kp = 75 Watts) or 600 kg/m/min (2 kp = 100 Watts)

The aim of the test is to elicit a HR of approximately 125-170 bpm. If, at the end of 6 min, HR has not reached the prescribed level, continue the test. Increase the resistance by 0.5 kp each minute until the participant attains an HR of at least 125 bpm.

6. Record the HR during the last 15 sec of each min.
7. Record the BP during the last 30 sec of each 2-min phase.
8. Refer to table 5.1 or 5.2 to obtain the maximal oxygen uptake (L/min) for the participant based on the average of the HRs in min 5 and 6.
9. Correct the value obtained from table 5.1 or 5.2 for age using the factor given in table 5.3.
10. After obtaining the absolute maximal oxygen uptake, determine the relative maximal oxygen uptake.
11. Refer to table 5.4 to determine the subject's fitness level.
12. For this and the following data-recording steps, use the Åstrand-Ryhming Data Collection Worksheet; at 0:45 into the stage, take and record HR.
13. At 1:30 into the stage, take and record BP and RPE.
14. At 1:45 into the stage, take and record HR.
15. At 2:45 into the stage, take and record HR.

16. At 3:30 into the stage, take and record BP and RPE.

17. At 3:45 into the stage, take and record HR.

18. At 4:45 into the stage, take and record HR.

19. At 5:30 into the stage, take and record BP and RPE.

20. At 5:45 into the stage, take and record HR.

21. Average the fifth and sixth HRs for a final HR.

22. Continue by performing either of the following substeps:

    a. If the participant has reached an average target HR of between 125 and 170 bpm, begin a 4-min cool-down stage. Record HR and BP after each minute. Talk with the participant about any problems that may have occurred. Refer to table 5.1 or table 5.2 to obtain the maximal oxygen uptake. Correct the value obtained for age using the correction factor given in table 5.3.

    b. If the participant has not reached an average target HR of between 125 and 170 bpm, continue the test for an additional minute, increasing the workload by 0.5 kp until the participant attains an HR of at least 125 bpm. Take and record HR, BP, and RPE at the end of the 1 min. Complete the test by following the procedures outlined in substep a.

YMCA Test

A portion of the following instructions for the YMCA test has been adapted, with permission, from Howley, E.T, and B.D. Franks. 2003. *Health Fitness Instructors' Handbook*, 4th ed. Champaign, IL: Human Kinetics.

1. Select a participant in your group to be the subject.

2. Complete the calculations for age-predicted maximum HR (HRmax) and target HR and record the participant's weight, age, resting HR, and BP.

3. Select the test protocol.

4. Estimate the participant's HRmax (220 – age = bpm).

5. Determine 85% of the participant's HRmax (HRmax × .85 = 85% HRmax) or 70% of HR reserve [(HRmax – resting HR) × (.70 + resting HR)].

6. Review the procedure with the participant. ("This is a two- to four-stage test, with each stage lasting 3 minutes. I will measure your heart rate during the last 15 to 30 seconds of minutes 2 and 3 of each stage, and I will measure your blood pressure and rate of perceived exertion during the last minute of each stage. If the two heart rate measurements I take in each stage are not within 6 beats per minute of each other, I will add time to the stage in 1-minute increments until your heart rate reaches a steady rate.")

7. Set and record the seat height (the participant should sit upright, and when the foot is at the bottom of the pedaling stroke, that leg should be slightly bent at the knee 5°).

8. Start the metronome (set at 100 bpm so that one foot is at the bottom of the pedaling stroke on each beat, resulting in 50 complete revolutions per minute).

9. Have the participant begin pedaling, with no resistance, in rhythm with the metronome. Continue this pace for 2-3 min for the participant to warm up.

10. As soon as the participant has maintained the warm-up pace for 2-3 min, set the resistance according to the protocol chosen.

11. Start the timer for the beginning of the stage. Check the resistance setting (it may drift) and observe the participant for signs or symptoms that require termination of the test. Continue until the participant reaches target HR. Here are some reminders and additional guidelines for the completion of each stage:

    a. If the two HRs obtained in the stage are within 6 bpm of each other (referred to as steady-state), increase the workload to the next stage according to the steady-state HR attained.

    b. If the HRs are not within 6 bpm of each other, continue the stage, measuring HR at the end of each additional minute until the participant achieves steady state, then increase the workload to the next stage according to the steady-state HR attained. See YMCA Protocol (page 50).

    c. Input the following data on the YMCA Data Collection Worksheet (page 139).

12. At 1:45 into the first stage, take and record HR.

13. At 2:30 into the first stage, take and record BP.

14. At 2:45 into the first stage, take and record HR and RPE.

15. Determine steady-state HR and increase the resistance (if necessary) outlined in the YMCA Protocol (page 50). Otherwise, proceed to step 27.

16. At 4:45 into the second stage, take and record HR.

17. At 5:30 into the second stage, take and record BP.

18. At 5:45 into the second stage, take and record HR and RPE.

19. Determine steady-state HR and increase to the resistance (if necessary) outlined in the YMCA Protocol Sheet. Otherwise, proceed to step 27.

20. At 7:45 into the third stage, take and record HR.

21. At 8:30 into the third stage, take and record BP.

22. At 8:45 into the third stage, take and record HR and RPE.

23. Determine steady-state HR and increase to the resistance (if necessary) outlined in the YMCA Protocol Sheet. Otherwise, proceed to step 27.

24. At 10:45 into the fourth stage, take and record HR.

25. At 11:30 into the fourth stage, take and record BP.

26. At 11:45 into the fourth stage, take and record HR and RPE.

27. Begin the cool-down by performing either of the following substeps:

a. Have the participant continue pedaling and reduce the resistance to a work rate equal to or less than that used in the first stage. Continue monitoring for at least 4 min of active recovery, taking HR and BP each minute.

b. If the participant is experiencing signs of discomfort or emergency symptoms, perform a passive cool-down (have the participant cease physical activity), monitoring the participant for at least 4 min and taking HR and BP each minute.

28. Plot the HRs obtained against the work rates from the last minute of each stage on the YMCA $\dot{V}O_2$max Estimation Graph (page 140). Then draw a line of best fit through the HRs up to the age-predicted HRmax. Draw a line straight down to estimate the work rate that would have been attained had the participant achieved HRmax. The value displayed is the estimated $\dot{V}O_2$max the participant would have achieved during a maximal stress test.

Arm Exercise Test Protocol

The arm exercise test is designed for people who are nonambulatory or those who perform dynamic upper-body work during occupational or recreational activities and are interested in assessing upper-body fitness. Be sure to gather the demographic and resting data described earlier (the date; the participant's name, age, resting HR, resting BP, age-predicted HRmax, and target HR) before testing.

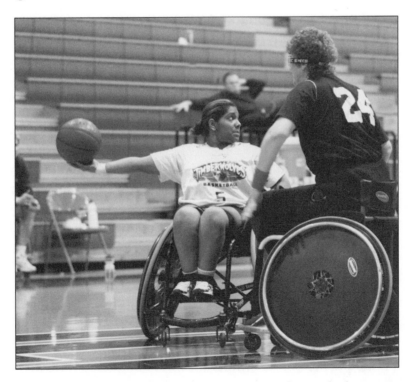

You should know how to use an arm ergometer, as it must be used when testing clients in wheelchairs or those with leg or foot injuries.

YMCA PROTOCOL

1. Set the first work rate at 150 kgm/min (0.5 kg at 50 rpm).

2. If the HR in the third minute of the first stage is

   a. <80, set the second stage at 750 kgm/min (2.5 kg at 50 rpm), set the third stage (if required) at 900 kgm/min (3.0 kg), and set the fourth stage (if required) at 1,050 kgm/min (3.5 kg).

   b. 80-89, set the second stage at 600 kgm/min (2.0 kg at 50 rpm), set the third stage (if required) at 750 kgm/min (3.0 kg), and set the fourth stage (if required) at 900 kgm/min (3.5 kg).

   c. 90-100, set the second stage at 450 kgm/min (1.5 kg at 50 rpm), set the third stage (if required) at 600 kgm/min (3.0 kg), and set the fourth stage (if required) at 750 kgm/min (3.5 kg).

   d. >100, set the second stage at 300 kgm/min (1.0 kg at 50 rpm), set the third stage (if required) at 450 kgm/min (3.0 kg), and set the fourth stage (if required) at 600 kgm/min (3.5 kg).

Note: kgm is also referred to as kpm.

Based on *The YMCA fitness assessment protocol,* 2000, edited by L.A. Golding (Champaign, IL: Human Kinetics).

Follow the steps below when using an arm exercise protocol.

1. Begin with no resistance on the flywheel; then increase 25 Watts (150 kg/m/min) every 2 min continuous stage without stopping (BP can be difficult to obtain), or

2. Begin with no resistance on the flywheel; then increase 25 Watts (150 kg/m/min) every 2 min discontinuous stage (better tolerated by participants and allows for more frequent, more reliable BP measures).

Factors to remember when assessing cardiorespiratory fitness with arm ergometry

- BP drops rapidly immediately after termination of upright arm-cranking exercise. Thus, an accurate measure of BP must be taken immediately.
- Maximal arm exercise $\dot{V}O_2$ is usually 70-80% of that determined from leg exercise.
- Values of HRmax are similar to or slightly lower than those achieved during treadmill or cycle ergometer exercise.

Discussion Questions

1. What is the purpose of determining cardiorespiratory fitness?
2. What is the most reliable and valid measure of cardiorespiratory fitness?
3. Why is it acceptable to use HR as a predictor of cardiorespiratory fitness?

4. What is the fitness classification of the participant being tested? (See table 5.1 for men and table 5.2 for women.)
5. What factors may affect the results of these predictions?
6. What are the determinants of oxygen uptake?
7. What are the objective criteria for terminating a maximal oxygen consumption test?

Bibliography

ACSM (American College of Sports Medicine). 2000. *ACSM's Guidelines for Exercise Testing and Prescription,* 6th ed. Baltimore: Lippincott Williams & Wilkins.

Borg, G. 1998. *Borg's Perceived Exertion and Pain Scales.* Champaign, IL: Human Kinetics.

Bruce, R.A., F. Kusumi, and D. Hosmer. 1973. Maximal oxygen intake and nomographic ssessment of functional aerobic impairment in cardiovascular disease. *American Heart Journal* 85: 545-62.

Howley, E.T., and B.D. Franks. 2003. *Health Fitness Instructor's Handbook,* 4th ed. Champaign, IL: Human Kinetics.

Montoye, H.J., T. Ayen, and R.A. Washburn. 1986. The estimation of $\dot{V}O_2$max from maximal and sub-maximal measurements in males, age 10-39. *Research Quarterly for Exercise and Sport* 57: 250-53.

Saltin, B., and P.O. Åstrand. 1967. Maximal oxygen uptake in athletes. *Journal of Applied Physiology* 23: 353-58.

TABLE 5.1

Prediction of Maximal Oxygen Uptake in Men From HR and Workload on a Cycle Ergometer

HR	300 kpm/min	600 kpm/min	900 kpm/min	1,200 kpm/min	1,500 kpm/min	HR	300 kpm/min	600 kpm/min	900 kpm/min	1,200 kpm/min	1,500 kpm/min
120	2.2	3.5	4.8			148		2.4	3.2	4.3	5.4
121	2.2	3.4	4.7			149		2.3	3.2	4.3	5.4
122	2.2	3.4	4.6			150		2.3	3.2	4.2	5.3
123	2.1	3.4	4.6			151		2.3	3.1	4.2	5.2
124	2.1	3.3	4.5	6.0		152		2.3	3.1	4.1	5.2
125	2.0	3.2	4.4	5.9		153		2.2	3.0	4.1	5.1
126	2.0	3.2	4.4	5.8		154		2.2	3.0	4.0	5.1
127	2.0	3.1	4.3	5.7		155		2.2	3.0	4.0	5.0
128	2.0	3.1	4.2	5.6		156		2.2	2.9	4.0	5.0
129	1.9	3.0	4.2	5.6		157		2.1	2.9	3.9	4.9
130	1.9	3.0	4.1	5.5		158		2.1	2.9	3.9	4.9
131	1.9	2.9	4.0	5.4		159		2.1	2.8	3.8	4.8
132	1.8	2.9	4.0	5.3		160		2.1	2.8	3.8	4.8
133	1.8	2.8	3.9	5.3		161		2.0	2.8	3.7	4.7
134	1.8	2.8	3.9	5.2		162		2.0	2.8	3.7	4.6
135	1.7	2.8	3.8	5.1		163		2.0	2.8	3.7	4.6
136	1.7	2.7	3.8	5.0		164		2.0	2.7	3.6	4.5
137	1.7	2.7	3.7	5.0		165		2.0	2.7	3.6	4.5
138	1.6	2.7	3.7	4.9		166		1.9	2.7	3.6	4.5
139	1.6	2.6	3.6	4.8		167		1.9	2.6	3.5	4.4
140	1.6	2.6	3.6	4.8	6.0	168		1.9	2.6	3.5	4.4
141		2.6	3.5	4.7	5.9	169		1.9	2.6	3.5	4.3
142		2.5	3.5	4.6	5.8	170		1.8	2.6	3.4	4.3
143		2.5	3.4	4.6	5.7						
144		2.5	3.4	4.5	5.7						
145		2.4	3.4	4.5	5.6						
146		2.4	3.3	4.4	5.6						
147		2.4	3.3	4.4	5.5						
148											
149											

The value should be corrected for age using the factor given in table 5.3.

Adapted, by permission, from P.O. Åstrand, 1960, "Aerobic work capacity in men and women with special references to age," *Acta Physiologica Scandanavia* 49 (suppl 169): 45-60.

TABLE 5.2

Prediction of Maximal Oxygen Uptake in Women From HR and Workload on a Cycle Ergometer

HR	300 kpm/ min	450 kpm/ min	600 kpm/ min	750 kpm/ min	900 kpm/ min	HR	300 kpm/ min	450 kpm/ min	600 kpm/ min	750 kpm/ min	900 kpm/ min
	2.6	3.4	4.1	4.8		148	1.6	2.1	2.6	3.1	3.6
	2.5	3.3	4.0	4.8		149		2.1	2.6	3.0	3.5
120	2.5	3.2	3.9	4.7		150		2.0	2.5	3.0	3.5
121	2.4	3.1	3.9	4.6		151		2.0	2.5	3.0	3.4
122	2.4	3.1	3.8	4.5		152		2.0	2.5	2.9	3.4
123	2.3	3.0	3.7	4.4		153		2.0	2.4	2.9	3.3
124	2.3	3.0	3.6	4.3		154		2.0	2.4	2.8	3.3
125	2.2	2.9	3.5	4.2		155		1.9	2.4	2.8	3.2
126	2.2	2.8	3.5	4.2	4.8	156		1.9	2.3	2.8	3.2
127	2.2	2.8	3.4	4.1	4.8	157		1.9	2.3	2.7	3.2
128	2.1	2.7	3.4	4.0	4.7	158		1.8	2.3	2.7	3.1
129	2.1	2.7	3.4	4.0	4.6	159		1.8	2.2	2.7	3.1
130	2.0	2.7	3.3	3.9	4.5	160		1.8	2.2	2.6	3.0
131	2.0	2.6	3.2	3.8	4.4	161		1.8	2.2	2.6	3.0
132	2.0	2.6	3.2	3.8	4.4	162		1.8	2.2	2.6	3.0
133	2.0	2.6	3.1	3.7	4.3	163		1.7	2.2	2.6	2.9
134	1.9	2.5	3.1	3.6	4.2	164		1.7	2.1	2.5	2.9
135	1.9	2.5	3.0	3.6	4.2	165		1.7	2.1	2.5	2.9
136	1.8	2.4	3.0	3.5	4.1	166		1.7	2.1	2.5	2.8
137	1.8	2.4	2.9	3.5	4.0	167		1.6	2.1	2.4	2.8
138	1.8	2.4	2.8	3.4	4.0	168		1.6	2.0	2.4	2.8
139	1.8	2.3	2.8	3.4	3.9	169		1.6	2.0	2.4	2.8
140	1.7	2.3	2.8	3.3	3.9	170		1.6	2.0	2.4	2.7
141	1.7	2.2	2.7	3.3	3.8						
142	1.7	2.2	2.7	3.2	3.8						
143	1.6	2.2	2.7	3.2	3.7						
144	1.6	2.2	2.6	3.2	3.7						
145	1.6	2.1	2.6	3.1	3.6						
146											
147											

The value should be corrected for age using the factor given in table 5.3.

Adapted, by permission, from P.O. Åstrand, 1960, "Aerobic work capacity in men and women with special references to age," *Acta Physiologica Scandanavia* 49 (suppl 169): 45-60.

TABLE 5.3

Correction Factors for Predicted Maximal Oxygen Uptake

Age	Factor	HRmax	Factor
15	1.10	210	1.12
25	1.00	200	1.00
35	0.87	190	0.93
40	0.83	180	0.83
45	0.78	170	0.75
50	0.75	160	0.69
55	0.71	150	0.64
60	0.68		
65	0.65		

Factor to be used for correction of predicted maximal oxygen uptake (a) when the participant is older than 30 to 35 yr of age, or (b) when the participant's maximal heart rate is known. Multiply the actual factor by the value obtained from table 5.1 or table 5.2.

Adapted, by permission, from P.O. Åstrand, 1960, "Aerobic work capacity in men and women with special references to age," *Acta Physiologica Scandanavia* 49 (suppl 169): 45-60

TABLE 5.4

Classification of Maximal Oxygen Uptake (Maximal Aerobic Power) by Age Group

Age	Low	Somewhat low	Average	High	Very high
Women					
20-29	≤1.69 ≤28	1.70-1.99 29-34	2.00-2.49 35-43	2.50-2.79 44-48	≥2.80 ≥49
30-39	≤1.59 ≤27	1.60-1.89 28-33	1.90-2.39 34-41	2.40-2.69 42-47	≥2.70 ≥48
40-49	≤1.49 ≤25	1.50-1.79 26-31	1.80-2.29 32-40	2.30-2.59 41-45	≥2.60 ≥46
50-65	≤1.29 ≤21	1.30-1.59 22-28	1.60-2.09 29-36	2.10-2.39 37-41	≥2.40 ≥42
Men					
20-29	≤2.79 ≤38	2.80-3.09 39-43	3.10-3.69 48-51	3.70-3.99 52-56	≥4.00 ≥57
30-39	≤2.49 ≤34	2.50-2.79 35-39	2.80-3.39 40-47	3.40-3.69 48-51	≥3.70 ≥52
40-49	≤2.19 ≤30	2.20-2.49 31-35	2.50-3.09 36-43	3.10-3.39 44-47	≥3.40 ≥48
50-59	≤1.89 ≤25	1.90-2.19 26-31	2.20-2.79 32-39	2.80-3.09 40-43	≥3.10 ≥44
60-69	≤1.59 ≤21	1.60-1.89 22-26	1.90-2.49 27-35	2.50-2.79 36-39	≥2.80 ≥40

The upper number, e.g., 1.69, refers to maximal oxygen uptake in L/min. The lower number, e.g., 28, refers to ml/kg – min. Weights used were 58 kg for females and 72 kg for males.

Adapted, by permission, from P.O. Åstrand, 1960, "Aerobic work capacity in men and women with special references to age," *Acta Physiologica Scandanavia* 49 (suppl 169): 45-60.

Assessment of Body Fat

PURPOSE

This lab exposes the student to field procedures commonly used to assess body fat. In addition, students will calculate results from the different equations used to determine body fat.

MATERIALS

1. Skinfold calipers
2. Gulick tape
3. Two copies of the BMI and Circumferential Sites Data Collection Worksheet and Classification (page 141)
4. Two copies of the Skinfold Sites Data Collection Worksheet and Classification (page 142)

Background Information

We know that a high amount of fat weight (obesity) is a risk factor for heart disease, diabetes, cancer, and other health problems (Howley and Franks 2003). Excess fat weight makes movement inefficient and difficult. A high lean body weight allows the body to accomplish work efficiently and expend more calories even at rest.

The term *body composition* refers to the percentage of body weight that is fat (% body fat) compared to total lean mass. Its measurement is based on the assumption that body weight can be divided into lean body weight and fat weight. Lean

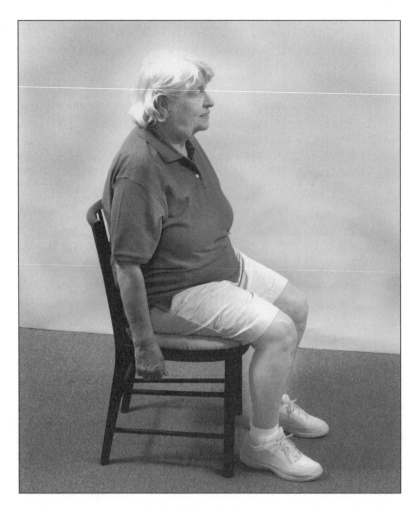

Being overweight can pose a serious health risk. Thus you must know how to assess percentage of body fat.

body mass encompasses all of the body's nonfat tissues, including the skeleton, water, muscle, connective tissue, organ tissues, and teeth. The fat component includes both the essential and nonessential fat stores. Essential fat includes fat incorporated into organs and tissues, with nonessential fat being primarily within adipose tissue. Evaluation of body composition typically is included as part of a health screening or physical fitness assessment.

Body composition can be measured in many ways, including both laboratory and field techniques. Although they are not as accurate, anthropometric methods provide a more practical and less expensive alternative than hydrostatic weighing to estimate body composition. Thus, this lab will focus on formulas and equations involving skinfolds, circumference, waist-to-hip ratio, and body mass index.

Interpreting Body Composition Data

It is important to distinguish between being *overweight* and being *overfat (obese)*. Overweight is defined as exceeding the normal or standard weight for a specific height and skeletal frame size, when grouped by gender. Being overweight is not necessarily undesirable, especially when the lean body mass is high. Measuring body density and calculating fat weight and lean body weight allow a more accurate method of estimating desired weight than using height-and-weight tables, which do not determine fat and lean weight. Overfat, or obesity, is defined as the state of having excess body fat. Although no universal agreement exists on the specific percentage of body fat that constitutes obesity, 25% body fat for men and 32% body fat for women are commonly used determinants. It is recommended that men and women maintain body fat percentages of 12-18% and 16-25%, respectively.

Interpretation of body composition must be individualized to each person. The exercise professional should be aware of the wide range of normal values and should not encourage all participants to achieve the same particular value. The principle of variability is important. Humans vary widely on any trait that can be measured, and body composition is no exception. The exercise professional must recognize this variability and take it into account in interpreting body composition data.

Anthropometric Definitions

• **Body mass index.** Body mass index (BMI), or Quetelet index, examines body weight relative to height. This index is calculated by dividing body weight (in kilograms) by height (in meters) squared (wt/ht^2). BMI is a good indicator of total body composition in population-based studies and is related to health outcomes. As BMI increases, mortality from heart disease, cancer, and diabetes also increases. Significant increases in risk begin at a BMI of about 27.8 kg/m^2 for men and 27.3 kg/m^2 for women.

• **Circumference.** Measurement of body girth may be reasonably accurate in estimating body fat (from prediction equations) in unfit subjects. These measurements, however, do not detect changes in body composition over time when lean tissue increases and fat mass decreases. Thus, for consistent evaluation of body fat percentage, they appear to be impractical.

• **Waist-to-hip ratio.** As mentioned earlier, excessive body fat is a health hazard. The distribution of body fat also affects a person's health. Levels of subcutaneous body fat in the upper body (waist measurement) and lower body (hip measurement) are distributed differently by gender, age, body type, and activity level. Fat in the abdomen (upper body) is associated with greater morbidity and mortality than is fat below the waist (lower body). Ideally, waist circumference should be smaller than hip circumference. Waist-to-hip ratios above .95 for men and .85 for women are considered to place the person at significantly increased risk for obesity-related health problems.

• **Skinfold.** Results from the skinfold method of estimating body composition correlate fairly well with hydrostatic weighing because approximately half of stored body fat is subcutaneous. Measuring the thickness of skinfolds involves grasping a fold of skin and fat and holding it away from the underlying muscle. The reliability of skinfold measurement depends on meticulous attention to detail in the techniques. Practice the techniques extensively and be precise in measuring at the exact anatomical locations indicated.

The values obtained from skinfold measurements can be used in several ways. We can total the values from several sites to arrive at the sum of skinfolds. We can use the sum of skinfolds to rank order individuals within a given group. We can also use the sum of skinfolds to evaluate body-fat changes following dietary restriction, exercise conditioning programs, or a combination of these. Skinfold measurements can also be used with mathematical equations to predict percentage of body fat. Keep in mind that equations derived from one segment of the population do a poor job of predicting percentage of fat for other populations; the equations are applicable only to groups similar in age and activity level to those from which the equations are derived. When the technicians performing the measurements are experienced and well trained, estimates of percentages body fat from skinfolds are generally within 3.7% of measurements obtained by using the underwater weighing technique.

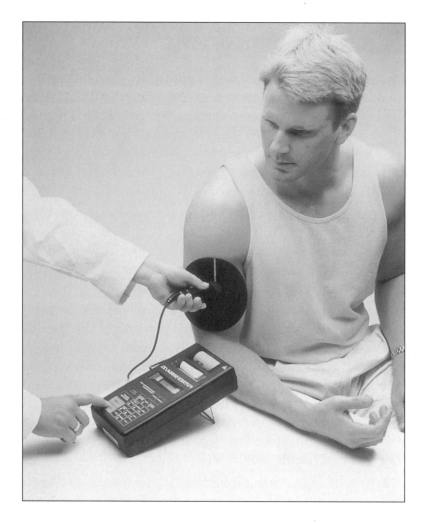

Because high-tech methods of body composition are often unavailable to the fitness professional, in this lab we will concentrate on more "hands-on" methods of body composition assessment.

Procedures

1. Follow the appropriate skinfold procedures (page 35) and circumferential technique (page 36) found in lab 4.

2. Collect skinfold measurements, circumferences, height, and weight for one male and one female in this lab.

3. Record the data on the data collection sheets for this lab.

4. Use appropriate anthropometric equations (male or female) from appendix E to calculate percentage body fat. Use the 7-site and both 3-site formulas.

5. Calculate a BMI and a waist-to-hip ratio using the data collected.

6. Determine the subjects' BMI classification according to table 6.1.

7. Determine each subject's fat mass and lean mass from each equation.

8. Determine each subject's body fat percentile and ranking according to table 6.2.

TABLE 6.1

Body Mass Index and Waist Circumference Disease Risk[†] Classification

		Waist circumference (men)		Waist circumference (women)	
		≤102 cm	≥102 cm	≤88 cm	≥88 cm
BMI	Classification	Risk level		Risk level	
<18.5	Underweight	...	...	...	...
18.5-24.9	Normal[§]	...	...	...	...
25.0-29.9	Overweight	Increased	High	Increased	High
30.0-34.9	Class 1 obesity	High	Very high	High	Very high
35.0-39.9	Class 2 obesity	Very high	Very high	Very high	Very high
≥40.0	Class 3 obesity	Extremely high	Extremely high	Extremely high	Extremely high

A gender-neutral value for waist circumference (>100 cm) has also been suggested as an index of obesity.

[†]Disease risk for type 2 diabetes, hypertension, and cardiovascular disease. Ellipses indicate no additional risk at these levels of BMI was assigned.

[§]Increased waist circumference can also be a marker for increased risk even in persons of normal weight.

Adapted, by permission, from American College of Sports Medicine, 2000, *ACSM's guidelines for exercise testing and prescription,* 6th ed. (Philadelphia, PA: Lippincott, Williams, and Wilkins), 64.

Discussion Questions

1. What are the similarities and differences among the different anthropometric measures discussed in this lab?

2. Which of the body composition assessment equations discussed in this lab are the most valid or reliable? Are there equations that are better or worse

TABLE 6.2

Body Composition Chart (Values Expressed in % Body Fat)

Percentile	Rating	Age (yr) 20-29	30-39	40-49	50-59	60+
Men						
90	Excellent	7.1	11.3	13.6	15.3	15.3
80		9.4	13.9	16.3	17.9	18.4
70	Good	11.8	15.9	18.1	19.8	20.3
60		14.1	17.5	19.6	21.3	22.0
50	Average	15.9	19.0	21.1	22.7	23.5
40		17.4	20.5	22.5	24.1	25.0
30	Poor	19.5	22.3	24.1	25.7	26.7
20		22.4	24.2	26.1	27.5	28.5
10	Extremely bad	25.9	27.3	28.9	30.3	31.2
Women						
90	Excellent	14.5	15.5	18.5	21.6	21.1
80		17.1	18.0	21.3	25.0	25.1
70	Good	19.0	20.0	23.5	26.6	27.5
60		20.6	21.6	24.9	28.5	29.3
50	Average	22.1	23.1	26.4	30.1	30.9
40		23.7	24.9	28.1	31.6	32.5
30	Poor	25.4	27.0	30.1	33.5	34.3
20		27.7	29.3	32.1	35.6	36.6
10	Extremely bad	32.1	32.8	35.0	37.9	39.3

Adapted, by permission, from American College of Sports Medicine, 2000, *ACSM's guidelines for exercise testing and prescription,* 6th ed. (Philadelphia, PA: Lippincott, Williams, and Wilkins), 67.

for specific age groups or populations? For what age groups and populations are these equations most appropriate?

3. What professional considerations are appropriate when using these measures in a field setting?

4. In procedure 4, you calculated body composition using the same data in different equations (7-site vs. 3-site). Compare the results from each equation. Do the results differ, and if so, why?

Bibliography

ACSM (American College of Sports Medicine). 1993. *ACSM's Resource Manual for Guidelines for Exercise Testing and Prescription,* 2nd ed. Philadelphia: Lea and Febiger.

ACSM (American College of Sports Medicine). 2000. *ACSM's Guidelines for Exercise Testing and Prescription*, 6th ed. Baltimore: Lippincott Williams, & Wilkins.

Howley, E.T., and B.D. Franks. 2003. *Health Fitness Instructor's Handbook*, 4th ed. Champaign, IL: Human Kinetics.

Evaluation of Muscular Strength and Endurance

PURPOSE

In this lab the student gains experience in administering assessments of muscular strength and endurance. The lab focuses on easily administered tests: one-repetition maximum (1 RM) for bench press (upper-body strength), 1 RM for seated leg press (lower-body strength), 1-min curl-up (crunch) for endurance, 1-min push-up for endurance, and grip strength.

MATERIALS

1. Stopwatch or clock with a second hand
2. Exercise mat
3. Handgrip dynamometer
4. Bench press and seated leg press
5. One copy of the Muscular Fitness Data Collection Worksheet and Classification (page 143)

Background Information

Muscular strength and endurance are very important components of fitness. Muscular strength is the ability to exert maximal force in a single muscular contraction, whereas muscular endurance is the ability to exert a submaximal force repeatedly over an extended period. Each of these components plays a unique role in activities of daily living and quality of life. Activities such as opening a jar, lifting a heavy milk jug from a grocery cart, or opening a heavy door all require muscular strength. Conversely, activities such as sweeping a floor, hammering a nail, and sawing a board all require a degree of muscular endurance. Through testing and evaluation an exercise professional may be able to identify weaknesses in strength and endurance that may need improvement. Evaluating these components also enables the exercise professional to determine the most appropriate course of action to improve a person's specific needs.

The Principle of Specificity

Training programs that emphasize exertion of force against a high resistance for a small number of repetitions enhance gains in strength; muscle size; and, to a lesser extent, endurance. These programs are appropriate for people who are already reasonably healthy and fit. Programs that emphasize a relatively low resistance and a high number of repetitions enhance muscular endurance and, to a smaller degree, strength and are more suited to clients or patients who are

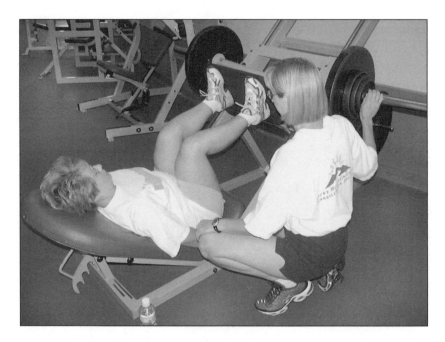

It is especially important that you monitor muscular strength and endurance when working with patients who have diseases that often cause muscle wasting, such as cancer.

significantly unfit. These examples illustrate the principle of *specificity of training*. Keep this principle in mind when administering strength tests. If participants are following an isotonic training program, they should be tested with isotonic strength tests to assess isotonic strength changes. The mode of testing should also be appropriate to the subject population being tested. For example, when you are assessing an older population with no previous weightlifting experience, a handgrip dynamometer test to assess upper-body strength is more appropriate than a 1 RM bench press test.

Definitions

Following is a list of terms and definitions that are often used when discussing muscular strength and endurance.

• **muscular strength**—The maximum amount of force that a muscle can exert in a single maximal effort.

• **muscular endurance**—The ability of a muscle to exert a submaximal force over a length of time.

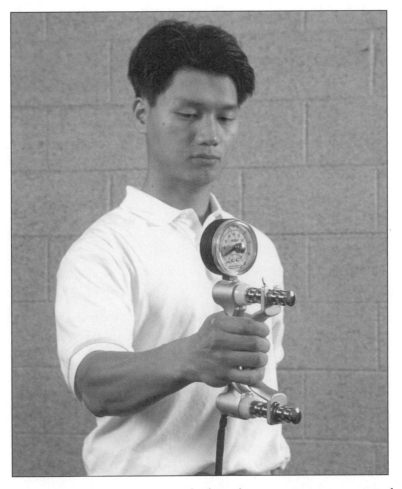

Your resistance training prescriptions must be based on accurate assessment of muscular strength and endurance.

- **isometric contraction**—A static muscle contraction wherein the overall length of the muscle does not change during the application of force against a fixed object.

- **isotonic contraction**—A dynamic muscle contraction in which the force remains constant. Isotonic exercises are typically performed with free weights or machines in which the resistance is "steered" along a fixed path. Accommodating resistance training (e.g., Nautilus, Cybex, etc.) is considered isotonic, although resistance is variable so that the lifter must exert maximum effort throughout the full range of motion.

- **isokinetic training**—Training that has both variable resistance and a speed-governing feature. Because isokinetic equipment controls the rate of contraction, it can potentially train the different types of muscle fiber.

- **Valsalva maneuver**—"Increased pressure in the abdominal and thoracic cavities caused by breath holding and extreme effort" (Howley and Franks 2003). Performing a Valsalva maneuver can inhibit the return of blood to the heart and increase blood pressure.

- **repetition maximum (1 RM)**—The maximum weight that a person can lift successfully for one repetition.

Procedures

Lab Activities

1. Each student should participate in all of the assessment procedures. Organize stations so that each lab group has an opportunity to participate in each assessment. The following assessment procedures are required:

    a. Bench press

    b. Leg press

    c. 1-min curl-up endurance

    d. 1-min push-up endurance

    e. Grip dynamometer

2. Follow the procedures for assessing muscular fitness and complete the Muscular Fitness Data Collection Worksheet and Classification, page 143, for one male and one female participant; use tables 7.1-7.5 to rate each participant.

Procedures for Assessing Muscular Fitness

The participant should not invoke the Valsalva maneuver during any of these exercises and should exhale during the concentric contraction phase of the bench press, leg press, push-up, and curl-up tests.

One-Repetition Maximum for Bench Press and Leg Press

The 1 RM tests assess upper-body strength (bench press) and lower body strength (leg press). Though the exercises are different, the steps for each are the same:

1. After a warm-up and familiarization with the equipment, start with a relatively low weight that the participant can easily and safely lift.

2. Add weight gradually until the participant can perform the lift correctly one time.

3. Encourage the participant to breathe freely with each lift.

4. Have the participant attempt to reach max within five trials with appropriate recovery, resting 1-2 min between trials (ACSM 2000).

TABLE 7.1

One-Repetition Maximum for Bench Press (Upper-Body Strength)

Percentile	Rating	Age (yr)				
		20-29	30-39	40-49	50-59	60+
Men						
90	Well above average	1.48	1.24	1.10	.97	.89
80		1.32	1.12	1.00	.90	.82
70	Above average	1.22	1.04	.93	.84	.77
60		1.14	.98	.88	.79	.72
50	Average	1.06	.93	.84	.75	.68
40		.99	.88	.80	.71	.66
30	Below average	.93	.83	.76	.68	.63
20		.88	.78	.72	.63	.57
10	Well below average	.80	.71	.65	.57	.53
Women						
90	Well above average	.90	.76	.71	.61	.64
80		.80	.70	.62	.55	.54
70	Above average	.74	.63	.57	.52	.51
60		.70	.60	.54	.48	.47
50	Average	.65	.57	.52	.46	.45
40		.59	.53	.50	.44	.43
30	Below average	.56	.51	.47	.42	.40
20		.51	.47	.43	.39	.38
10	Well Below Average	.48	.42	.38	.37	.33

Adapted, by permission, from American College of Sports Medicine, 2000, *ACSM's guidelines for exercise testing and prescription*, 6th ed. (Philadelphia, PA: Lippincott, Williams, and Wilkins), 82.

TABLE 7.2

One-Repetition Maximum for Leg Press (Lower-Body Strength)

Percentile	Rating	Age (yr)				
		20-29	30-39	40-49	50-59	60+
Men						
90	Well above average	2.20	2.07	1.92	1.80	1.73
80		2.13	1.93	1.82	1.71	1.62
70	Above average	2.05	1.85	1.74	1.64	1.56
60		1.97	1.77	1.68	1.58	1.49
50	Average	1.91	1.71	1.62	1.52	1.43
40		1.83	1.65	1.57	1.46	1.38
30	Below average	1.74	1.59	1.51	1.39	1.30
20		1.63	1.52	1.44	1.32	1.25
10	Well below average	1.51	1.43	1.35	1.22	1.16
Women						
90	Well above average	1.82	1.61	1.48	1.37	1.32
80		1.68	1.47	1.37	1.25	1.18
70	Above average	1.58	1.39	1.29	1.17	1.13
60		1.50	1.33	1.23	1.10	1.04
50	Average	1.44	1.27	1.18	1.05	.99
40		1.37	1.21	1.13	.99	.93
30	Below average	1.27	1.15	1.08	.95	.88
20		1.22	1.09	1.02	.88	.85
10	Well below average	1.14	1.00	.94	.78	.72

Adapted, by permission, from American College of Sports Medicine, 2000, *ACSM's guidelines for exercise testing and prescription*, 6th ed. (Philadelphia, PA: Lippincott, Williams, and Wilkins), 83.

One-Minute Curl-Up (Crunch) Endurance (Muscular Endurance for Abdomen)

1. The participant should assume a supine position on the floor with knees bent so that the heels are positioned approximately 18 in. from the buttocks. The arms are held at the side, with a strip of masking tape placed on the floor at the fingertips. Place a second strip of tape exactly 8 cm (age ≥45 yr) or 12 cm (age <45 yr) beyond the first strip (toward your heels).

2. The participant does slow, controlled curl-ups, lifting the shoulder blades off the mat and returning to the start position after each repetition. To successfully complete a repetition, the participant should touch the fingertips to the second strip of masking tape, with the trunk making a 30-degree angle with the mat and the low back flattened before each curl-up. Remind the participant to be sure to keep the neck straight; curving the neck can cause injury.

TABLE 7.3

One-Minute Curl-Up (Crunch) Abdominal Endurance

Percentile	Rating	Age (yr) 20-29	30-39	40-49	50-59	60+
Men						
90	Well above average	75	75	75	74	53
80		56	69	75	60	33
70	Above average	41	46	67	45	26
60		31	36	51	35	19
50	Average	27	31	39	27	16
40		24	26	31	23	9
30	Below average	20	19	26	19	6
20		13	13	21	13	0
10	Well below average	4	0	13	0	0
Women						
90	Well above average	70	55	50	48	50
80		45	43	42	30	30
70	Above average	37	34	33	23	24
60		32	28	28	16	19
50	Average	27	21	25	9	13
40		21	15	20	2	9
30	Below average	17	12	14	0	3
20		12	0	5	0	0
10	Well below average	5	0	0	0	0

Adapted, by permission, from American College of Sports Medicine, 2000, *ACSM's guidelines for exercise testing and prescription*, 6th ed. (Philadelphia, PA: Lippincott, Williams, and Wilkins), 86

3. At the "go" signal from you, the participant should perform as many curl-ups as possible in 1 min. Score the test as the number of correctly performed curl-ups completed in the 1-min period allotted. (ACSM 2000).

One Minute Push-Up Endurance

1. Male participants perform this test in the standard position (on toes) and females in the modified position (on knees).

2. The participant must lower the body until the chin touches the mat. The abdomen should not touch the mat.

3. Remind the participant to keep the back straight at all times and to push up to a straight-arm position.

4. Score this test as the maximum number of push-ups performed consecutively without rest (Golding, Myers, and Sinning 1991).

TABLE 7.4

One-Minute Push-Up Endurance

Percentile	Rating	Age (yr)				
		20-29	30-39	40-49	50-59	60+
Men						
90	Well above average	41	32	25	24	24
80		34	27	21	17	16
70	Above average	30	24	19	14	11
60		27	21	16	11	10
50	Average	24	19	13	10	9
40		21	16	12	9	7
30	Below average	18	14	10	7	6
20		16	11	8	5	4
10	Well below average	11	8	5	4	2
Women						
90	Well above average	32	31	28	23	25
80		26	24	22	17	15
70	Above average	22	21	18	13	12
60		20	17	14	10	10
50	Average	16	14	12	9	6
40		14	12	10	5	4
30	Below average	11	10	7	3	2
20		9	7	4	1	-
10	Well below average	5	4	2	-	-

Adapted, by permission, from American College of Sports Medicine, 2000, *ACSM's guidelines for exercise testing and prescription,* 6th ed. (Philadelphia, PA: Lippincott, Williams, and Wilkins), 85.

Grip Dynamometer Test

1. The person being tested should chalk or dry the hands before the test to ensure a firm grasp on the instrument.

2. The participant holds the handgrip between the palm at the base of the thumb and the second joint of the fingers.

3. The participant holds the grip dynamometer out in front of the body and is allowed to move the body when actually squeezing.

4. The participant should squeeze the dynamometer with maximum effort.

5. Perform two trials with the participant using the dominant hand, with a 1-2-min rest period between trials. Record the better of the trials for comparison to norms (Montoye and Lamphier 1977).

TABLE 7.5

Standard Values for Grip Strength—Dominant Hand (kg)

Percentile	Rating	Age (yr)				
		20-29	30-39	40-49	50-59	60+
Men						
90	Well above average	>54	>53	>51	>49	>49
70	Above average	51-54	50-53	48-51	46-49	46-49
50	Average	43-50	43-49	41-47	39-45	39-45
30	Below average	39-42	39-42	37-40	35-38	35-38
10	Well below average	<39	<39	<37	<35	<35
Women						
90	Well above average	>36	>36	>35	>33	>33
70	Above average	33-36	34-36	33-35	31-33	31-33
50	Average	26-32	28-33	27-32	25-30	25-30
30	Below average	22 – 25	25 - 27	24 – 26	22 - 24	22 – 24
10	Well below average	<22	<25	<24	<22	<22

Adapted, by permission, from T. Ishiko, 1975, The organism and muscular work. In *Fitness, health, and work capacity: International standards for assessment,* edited by L.A. Larson (Upper Saddle River, New Jersey: Addison Wesley), 61.

Discussion Questions

1. Why is it important to choose the appropriate type of assessment technique?
2. Describe isokinetic strength and endurance training and the type of equipment it requires.
3. What is the level of strength and endurance of the persons on whom you have collected data? Are there any areas in which these participants need to improve?
4. What are the benefits and drawbacks of the grip dynamometer test?
5. Why do fitness professionals often examine abdominal endurance?

Bibliography

ACSM (American College of Sports Medicine). 2000. *ACSM's Guidelines for Exercise Testing and Prescription,* 6th ed. Baltimore: Lippincott Williams & Wilkins.

Golding, J.A., C.R. Myers, and W.E. Sinning. 1991. *The Y's Way to Fitness.* Chicago: National Board of YMCA.

Howley, E.T., and B.D. Franks. 2003. *Health Fitness Instructors Handbook,* 4th ed. Champaign, IL: Human Kinetics.

Montoye, H.J., and D.K. Lamphier. 1977. Grip and arm strength in males and females age 10-59. *Research Quarterly for Exercise Science and Sport* 48: 109.

Evaluation of Flexibility

PURPOSE

This lab familiarizes the student with the different tests used to evaluate flexibility. Six tests (the ankle flexibility test, shoulder elevation test, trunk extension test, sit-and-reach test, Thomas test, and straight-leg-raise test) will be presented.

MATERIALS

1. Goniometer
2. Sit-and-reach box
3. Yardstick or meter stick
4. Three copies of the Flexibility Data Collection Worksheet and Classification (page 145)
5. Mat or table

Background Information

Flexibility refers to the ability to move the body parts through a wide range of motion without undue strain to the articulations and muscle attachments. Maintaining a reasonable degree of flexibility is necessary for efficient body movement. Being flexible and lithe may also decrease the chances of sustaining muscle injury or soreness and low back pain. Proper muscle balance, in which agonist and antagonist muscle pairs maintain appropriate ratios of strength, flexibility, and length to one another, is important for avoiding musculoskeletal injury. Flexibility assessment and exercises are crucial for lengthening muscles that are too tight.

Muscle Injury and Soreness

To move body segments, the muscles opposite those performing the movement (antagonist muscles) must lengthen sufficiently. Tight muscles, tendons, and ligaments limit lengthening of the antagonist muscles and thus reduce the range of movement of body segments. Soreness or injury may result when tight muscles are subjected to strenuous physical activity.

Low Back Pain

Low back pain is one of the most common complaints among adults in the United States. Low back problems

- account for more lost work hours than any other type of occupational injury, and
- are the most frequent cause of activity limitation in people under 45 yr of age in the United States.

Muscular deficiencies, including lack of abdominal strength, have been recognized as important considerations in physical medicine regimens to treat back pain. The abdominal muscles play a major role in preventing excessive anterior or forward tilt of the pelvis, and strong abdominal musculature appears to play a very important role in supporting the trunk in postures often considered compromising to the lower back. In forward-leaning postures, strong abdominal muscle contraction can appreciably increase intra-abdominal pressure; this appears to create a splinting-like effect on the trunk, which in turn decreases the stress placed on intervertebral discs.

Two groups of antagonist muscles (the hip flexors and the hip extensors) are also associated with low back pain; the former tilts the pelvis anteriorly and the latter tilts the pelvis posteriorly. Here the concern is lack of extensibility or too much tightness in the pelvis rather than lack of strength. Extreme shortening of either group can have a deleterious effect on the functioning of the lower back (Howley and Franks 2002).

Measuring Flexibility

Flexibility measurements include flexion and extension movements. No general test is available that provides representative values of total body flexibility; tests are specific to each joint and muscle group and area of connective tissue. Because flexibility is joint specific, determining the range of motion of a few joints does not necessarily provide an indicator of flexibility in other joints.

The most accurate tests of flexibility are those in which a goniometer is used to measure the actual degrees of rotation of the various joints. A goniometer is a protractor type of instrument used to measure the joint angle at both extremes in the total range of movement. The goniometer has two arms that attach to two body parts, with the center of the instrument over the exact center of the joint tested (ACSM 1993).

Procedures

General Instructions

1. Evaluate three of your classmates using the following flexibility tests:
   a. Ankle flexibility test
   b. Shoulder elevation test
   c. Trunk extension test
   d. Sit-and-reach test
   e. Thomas test
   f. Straight-leg-raise test

2. Record your results on the Flexibility Data Collection Worksheet and Classification (page 145).

Flexibility Tests

Following are the instructions and tables (tables 8.1-8.4) necessary for performing the required flexibility tests. Because hip flexors and hip extensors play a critical role in supporting a person's posture and avoiding low back discomfort, assessing flexibility of these muscle groups is important. Therefore, we have included two simple tests that can provide information about the flexibility of these muscle groups.

Ankle Flexibility Test

The ankle flexibility test measures a person's ability to flex and extend the ankle.

1. In preparation for the test, emphasize a brief warm-up of gradual ankle movements to increase the safety of the test and give the highest measurements possible.

2. The participant sits on a flat surface, with the back of the knee touching the surface. The tester crouches or sits at the participant's side. Keeping the heel on the ground, the participant pulls the foot in toward the body (dorsiflexed) as much as possible, keeping toes straight.

3. Measure this angle by aligning a protractor or goniometer with the anklebone and the side of the leg; record this angle. Then have the participant extend the foot (plantar flex) in the other direction as far as possible; record the angle of this foot position.

TABLE 8.1

Standard Values for Ankle Flexibility

Percentile	Rating	Ankle flexibility score (degrees of movement)
Men		
90	Well above average	77-99
70	Above average	63-76
50	Average	48-62
30	Below average	34-47
10	Well below average	15-33
Women		
90	Well above average	81-89
70	Above average	68-80
50	Average	56-67
30	Below average	43-55
10	Well below average	32-42

Adapted, from B.L. Johnson and J.K. Nelson, 1969, *Practical measurements for evaluation in physical education,* 4th ed. (Minneapolis, MN: Burgess Publishing). By permission of author.

4. The difference between the positions of dorsiflexion and plantar flexion is the average flexibility score in degrees of movement.

5. Repeat the test two more times (ACSM 1993). Record the best score on the worksheet.

Shoulder Elevation Test

This test assesses the flexibility of the muscles in the front of the chest and shoulders (pecs and anterior deltoids).

1. The participant stands with arms relaxed and hands pronated (knuckles facing forward) and grasps a yardstick or meter stick in the hands across the front of the body. The tester measures the arm length from the acromion process to the top of the stick (proximal edge) (figure 8.1*a*).

2. Next, the participant assumes a prone position lying on the floor with the chin touching the floor and the arms overhead, hands still holding the stick. Have the participant slowly raise the stick as high as possible while keeping the chin on the floor and the elbows extended. Measure the distance in inches from the floor to the bottom of the stick (figure 8.1*b*). Repeat the test two more times.

3. Calculate flexibility: Multiply the greatest height measured by 100 and divide this value by the arm length (ACSM 1993).

$$\text{flexibility} = \frac{\text{best trial (in.)} \times 100 \text{ arm}}{\text{length (in.)}}$$

TABLE 8.2

Standard Values for Shoulder Elevation

Percentile	Rating	Shoulder elevation score (in.)
Men		
90	Well above average	106-123
70	Above average	88-105
50	Average	70-87
30	Below average	53-69
10	Well below average	35-52
Women		
90	Well above average	105-123
70	Above average	86-104
50	Average	68-85
30	Below average	50-67
10	Well below average	31-49

Adapted, from B.L. Johnson and J.K. Nelson, 1969, *Practical measurements for evaluation in physical education,* 4th ed. (Minneapolis, MN: Burgess Publishing). By permission of author.

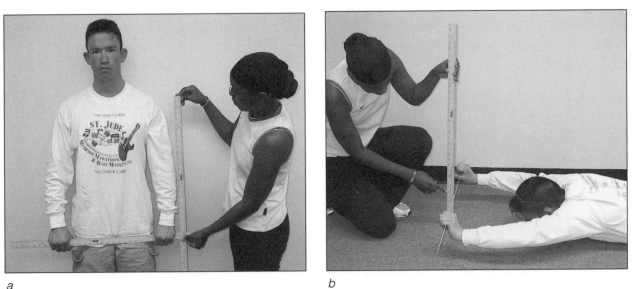

a *b*

FIGURE 8.1 Be sure the participant's arms are relaxed and that his hands are pronated when you take the preliminary measurement for the shoulder extension test *(a)*. As the participant raises his or her arms be sure that the elbows are extended and the chin remains in contact with the floor *(b)*.

Trunk Extension Test

This test assesses the flexibility of the muscles in the abdominal region.

1. Caution: People with existing or suspected back problems should not attempt this test because the motion involved exerts pressure on the posterior area of the lumbar vertebrae. Make sure participants stretch before beginning the test.

2. First measure trunk length by having the participant sit back against a wall with legs extended out forward. Place the yardstick in front of the participant, between the legs, to make it easier to see the number for a more accurate reading. Trunk length is defined as the vertical distance (in in.) between the floor and the suprasternal notch.

3. After taking this measurement, have the participant lie on his or her stomach and place the hands on the lower back. A second person holds the participant's feet and hips to the floor while the participant slowly hyperextends the back as far up and back as possible. The tester records the vertical distance (in in.) between the mat and the suprasternal notch (figure 8.2). Repeat the test two more times (ACSM 1993).

4. Calculate trunk extension:

trunk extension = best trial (in.) × 100 trunk length (in.)

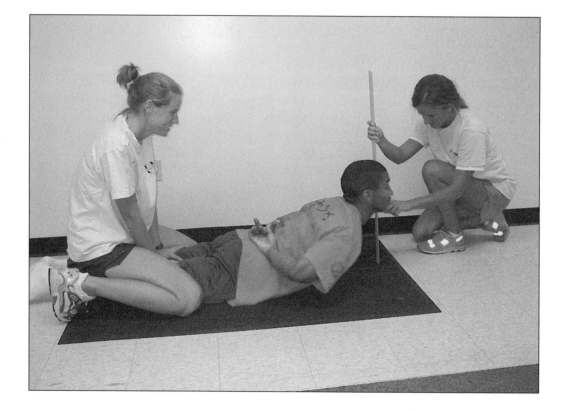

FIGURE 8.2　Trunk extension technique.

TABLE 8.3

Standard Values for Trunk Extension

Percentile	Rating	Trunk extension score (in.)
Men		
90	Well above average	50-64
70	Above average	43-49
50	Average	37-42
30	Below average	31-36
10	Well below average	28-30
Women		
90	Well above average	48-63
70	Above average	42-47
50	Average	35-41
30	Below average	29-34
10	Well below average	23-28

Adapted, from B.L. Johnson and J.K. Nelson, 1969, *Practical measurements for evaluation in physical education,* 4th ed. (Minneapolis, MN: Burgess Publishing). By permission of author.

Sit-and-Reach Test

This test assesses the flexibility of the low back and hip joint.

1. Caution: To avoid the potentially negative effects of blood flow limitations to the heart and increases in blood pressure, the participant should not invoke the Valsalva maneuver and should breathe easily during the exercise.

2. The participant should perform a short warm-up before you administer this test. It is also recommended that the participant avoid fast, jerky movements, which may increase the possibility of injury. Have the participant remove shoes.

3. Place a yardstick on the floor and apply tape across it at a right angle to the 15-in. mark. The participant sits with the yardstick between the legs, with legs extended at right angles to the taped line on the floor. Heels should touch the edge of the taped line and be about 10-12 in. apart. If a standard sit-and-reach box is available, have the participant place the heels against the edge of the box.

4. The participant slowly reaches forward as far as possible with both hands on the yardstick, holding this position momentarily. Be sure that the participant keeps the hands parallel and does not stretch or lead with one hand. The fingertips of one hand can overlap those of the other, and the hands should be in contact

with the yardstick or measuring portion of the sit-and-reach box (see figure 8.3). Suggest that the participant exhale and drop the head between the arms when reaching. The tester should make sure the participant keeps the knees straight, however, do not press them down (ACSM 2000).

5. The score is the most distant point (in inches) that the fingertips reach on the yardstick. Record the best of three trials.

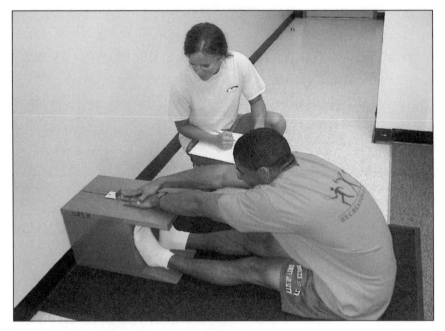

FIGURE 8.3   The sit-and-reach test.

TABLE 8.4

Standard Values for Trunk Flexion (in Inches)

Percentile	Rating	Age 20-29	30-39	40-49	50-59	60+
Men						
90	Well above average	>21	>20	>19	>18	>17
70	Above average	19-21	18-20	17-19	16-18	15-17
50	Average	13-18	12-17	11-16	10-15	9-14
30	Below average	10-12	9-11	8-10	7-9	6-8
10	Well below average	<10	<9	<8	<7	<6
Women						
90	Well above average	>23	>22	>21	>20	>19
70	Above average	22-23	21-22	20-21	19-20	18-19
50	Average	16-21	15-20	14-19	13-18	12-17
30	Below average	13-15	12-14	11-13	10-12	9-11
10	Well below average	<13	<12	<11	<10	<9

Based on *Y's way to physical fitness,* 3rd ed., 1989, edited by L.A. Golding, C. Myers, and W.E. Sinning (Champaign, IL: Human Kinetics).

Thomas Test

The Thomas test assesses the flexibility of the hip flexors.

1. Have the participant lie on his or her back.

2. The participant brings one leg (the contralateral leg, or the leg that is not being tested) in the direction of the chest just to the point where the lumbar spine is snug to the floor or table.

3. If the tested leg remains in contact with the floor or table during this maneuver, the hip flexors of that leg are adequately flexible.

4. If the tested leg rises, its hip flexors are likely to be inflexible (short) (Howley and Franks 2003).

5. Record whether the hip flexors in the right and left legs are flexible or inflexible on the Flexibility Data Collection Worksheet and Classification (page 145).

Straight-Leg-Raise Test

The straight-leg-raise test assesses the flexibility of the hip extensors.

1. Have the participant lie on his or her back.

2. Be sure the low back is snug against the floor or table (posteriorly rotated).

3. The tester raises one of the participant's legs while ensuring that the other leg remains extended and flat on the floor or table.

4. Measure the angle of flexion (range of motion) with (a) a goniometer by placing its axis on the greater trochanter or (b) an inclinometer placed just below the tibial tubercle.

5. A minimum angle of 80 degrees is acceptable for this passive straight-leg raise.

6. An angle of 90 degrees is desirable (Howley and Franks 2003)

7. Record the angle on the Flexibility and Data Collection Worksheet and Classification. In addition, report whether the range of motion is acceptable or unacceptable.

Discussion Questions

1. Compare the results of the three classmates you tested against the norms.

2. Summarize the six flexibility tests done in this lab. Can they be used to evaluate overall flexibility? Why or why not?

3. How is flexibility or lack of flexibility related to low back pain?

4. What can you do to improve the flexibility of your clients (i.e., what specific exercises can you recommend)?

Bibliography

ACSM (American College of Sports Medicine). 1993. *ACSM's Resource Manual for Guidelines for Exercise Testing and Prescription,* 2d ed. Philadelphia: Lea & Febiger.

ACSM (American College of Sports Medicine). 2000. *ACSM's Guidelines for Exercise Testing and Prescription,* 6th ed. Baltimore: Lippincott Williams & Wilkins.

Howley, E.T., and B.D. Franks. 2003. *Health Fitness Instructor's Handbook,* 4th ed. Champaign, IL: Human Kinetics.

ECG Placement and Monitor Operations

PURPOSE

This lab provides opportunities for students to gain experience in locating for placement, preparing for placement, and placing the 10 electrodes used in a 12-lead electrocardiogram (ECG). In addition, it describes the operations of the monitor, and you will have an opportunity to utilize all the operations.

MATERIALS

1. Protective gloves
2. Gauze and alcohol prep pads
3. Dry-shave razors
4. Electrodes
5. Towel(s)
6. Laundry bag
7. Disinfectant soap
8. Biohazard waste bag
9. Biohazard sharps bag

10. 10% bleach solution
11. Voltmeter
12. ECG monitor with paper
13. Lab coat
14. Scissors

Background Information

Electrocardiography is the science of monitoring the electrical function of the heart. The machine used to determine function is called an electrocardiograph, which records an electrocardiogram (ECG). An ECG is an electrical record of the current flowing through the heart muscle during the depolarization and repolarization of a contraction (Dubin 1990).

Procedures

Practice Procedures

Following are the overall instructions for this lab along with the step-by-step procedures for ECG preparation and placement and conducting an ECG.

Summary of Procedures for Lab 9

1. Locate, prep, and place electrodes on your lab partner.
2. Locate electrode placements on at least three other lab partners.
3. After placing the electrodes, place the label leads from the ECG on the appropriate electrodes.
4. Be sure that you can monitor every lead without artifact (irrelevant or unwanted information).
5. Calculate HR for each ECG in your group.
    a. The electrical activity of the heart is represented on an ECG by a series of up-and-down deflections, or waves. The labels given to each deflection correspond to the letters P, Q, R, S, and T. One heartbeat on an ECG is represented by the P-QRS-T complex. The QRS represents the depolarization of the ventricles. Count the number of QRS complexes in a 6-sec period (two sequential 3-sec periods using the 3-sec marks) and multiply by 10.
    b. The following numbers represent the calculated HR when two sequential R peaks are 1 small box (.4 sec), 2 small boxes, or 3 small boxes apart in distance: 300, 150, and 100, respectively. Furthermore,

the calculated HR for when two sequential R peaks are 4 small boxes, 5 small boxes, and 6 small boxes apart in distance is 75, 60, and 50, respectively. This is referred to as the triplicate technique for determining HR.

 c. Count the number of tiny boxes between two successive R peaks and divide by 1,500.

Steps for ECG Prep and Placement

Never place an ECG electrode on a bony area; otherwise the monitor will pick up artifact, potentially resulting in irregular ECG recordings.

1. Obtain a lab coat and properly fitting protective gloves.

2. Set out the equipment needed to prep the subject for the ECG.

3. Give the participant verbal instructions:

 a. "My name is _____, and I will be preparing you for an ECG."

 b. "I will have to shave a few areas on the chest and rough up the area in order for the electrodes to have a good contact surface for adherence."

 c. "The electrodes are necessary so that we can monitor the electrical activity of the heart during the test."

 d. "A good contact surface will augment the monitor's ability to pick up the heart rate and also prevent the electrodes from falling off during the testing procedures."

 e. "The rubbing with the gauze may cause some mild skin irritation, but this should subside within two days."

 f. "Do you have any questions?"

4. Following are the technician instructions for ECG preparation.

 a. Have the participant lie supine on the prep table with the left side of the chest nearer the technician.

 b. Mark the 10 areas (4 limb leads and 6 chest leads) to be shaved (see figure 9.1).

 c. Begin shaving the areas for electrode placement on the limb lead areas first. Use discretion with female clients.

- Use a long stroke with the dry-shave razor.
- If the subject has a lot of hair, it is acceptable to trim the hair first with scissors.
- It may be necessary to dip the razor in a small container of water to rid the blades of excess hair.
- Place the used dry-shave razor in the biohazard sharps container.

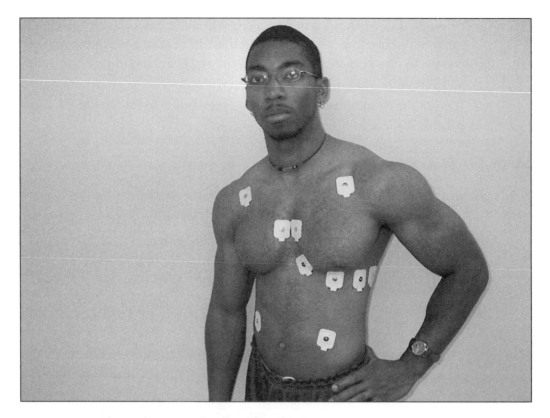

FIGURE 9.1   The 10 locations for electrode placement.

d. Shave the correct anatomical places.

- Shave the locations for the right arm (RA) and left arm (LA) leads in the hollow space below the clavicle and the medial edge of the shoulder.

- Shave the right leg (RL) and left leg (LL) lead locations approximately 1 in. above the navel below the rib cage on each side of the trunk.

- From the clavicle, count down with your fingers to the fourth intercostal.

- At this point, shave the V_1 and V_2 places (refer to figure 9.1).

- The next space to be shaved on the chest is V_4, which is to be placed directly below the nipple (mid clavicular) in the fifth intercostal space. The electrode should not be placed on breast tissue. If the placement must be moved from the specified location, this should be reported on the ECG strip.

- V_3 should then be shaved, midway between V_2 and V_4.

- V_6 is the next space to be shaved, in the mid axillary region under the left arm in the fifth intercostal space and horizontal to V_4.

- Finally, V_5 should be shaved, placed midway between V_4 and V_6 (anterior axillary) (ACSM 2000).

e. Rub all the shaved areas with gauze and alcohol.

- Either soak the gauze with alcohol and rub, thus roughing up and cleansing the area simultaneously, or rub the area with plain gauze to rough it up and then apply an alcohol prep pad to cleanse it.
- The area that has been rubbed and cleansed should be visibly red or pink.
- Place the gauze and alcohol prep pads in the biohazard waste bag.
- Follow the same directions for preparing the six chest lead sites.

f. Place the limb lead electrodes on the chest first. The limb leads will allow the technicians to view the heart through leads I, II, III, AVR, AVL, and AVF (Dubin 1990).

g. Next, place the chest lead electrodes on the chest.

h. Use the voltmeter to determine the conductivity of the electrode.

- Place the black probe on the ground electrode (RL) and move the red probe around to the other electrodes.
- Look for voltmeter readings of 600 mega-ohms or higher.
- If the voltmeter readings are too low, it may be necessary to reapply the electrode after additional rubbing and cleansing of the area.

5. Follow proper cleanup procedures.

a. Make sure all gauze and alcohol pads are discarded in the biohazard waste bags.

b. Make certain the dry-shave razor is properly discarded in the biohazard sharps container.

c. Spray the 10% bleach solution on the prep table after completing testing of each participant, and discard the towel in the laundry basket.

d. Remove the latex gloves and discard them in the biohazard waste bag.

e. Wash your hands with disinfectant soap after completing testing of each participant.

Electrocardiograph Monitor and Operations

The ECG monitor (figure 9.2) will provide you with a real-time presentation of the electrical activity in the heart and a hard copy for record keeping. Various models of ECG monitors have unique features.

Steps for Conducting an ECG

1. Prepare the monitor.

a. Turn on the power for the electrocardiograph on the lower left-hand side of the machine.

b. Turn on the power to the monitor by pushing the red button in the lower center of the monitor.

c. Place the gray cable, with the leads, into the electrocardiograph. Place the end of the cord into the lower right-hand side of the electrocardiograph, which is located in the front.

d. Make sure the 000 button on the electrocardiograph has been pushed, because the leads have not been hooked to the participant being tested.

e. Check the ECG paper supply by lifting the gray chrome plate located on top of the electrocardiograph. The plate will slide up, allowing you to see the paper. Paper supply is low if red streaks appear on the ECG strip. Change the roll if necessary.

f. Manually unroll approximately 12 in. of the roll and slide the chrome plate back into place.

g. Press the AUTO RUN button, which will automatically line up the ECG paper roll.

h. Make sure the paper speed is set to 25 mm per sec.

- The paper grid provides for a determination of duration of time (horizontal measurement); small block equals .04 sec; large block equals .20 sec. The 3-sec markers, of course, indicate 3 sec of elapsed time.

- The paper grid also provides for a determination of amplitude or voltage (vertical measure). This measurement is made in millimeters (mm), with each small box representing 1 mm on the vertical axis above or below the isoelectric line (baseline; no electrical activity).

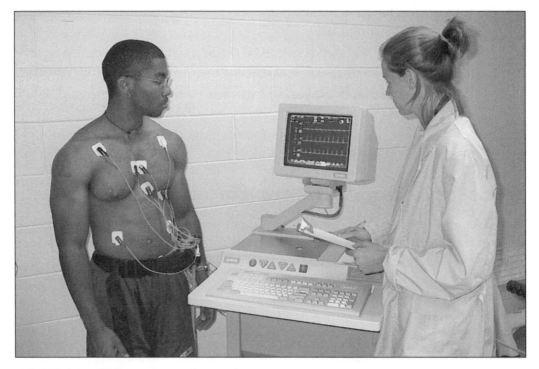

FIGURE 9.2   ECG monitor and operations.

2. Administer the ECG using the following procedures.

   a. Have the participant lie supine on the prep table with the left side closer to the technician.

   b. The participant should lie still with arms at sides and legs uncrossed.

   c. Rest the box of leads on the participant's abdomen.

   d. Begin placing the labeled leads on the corresponding electrodes on the chest.

3. Check the integrity of the leads by checking the monitor.

   a. Press the 1,2,3 button. Check the monitor.

   b. Press the R,L,F button. Check the monitor.

   c. Press the $V_{1,2,3}$ button. Check the monitor.

   d. Press the $V_{4,5,6}$ button. Check the monitor.

   e. If artifact is present, it may be necessary to check and replace the lead that is displaying artifact.

   f. If everything is in order, have the participant lie still with no muscular movement.

4. Record an ECG.

   a. Press the AUTO RUN button, which will automatically record an ECG for all 12 leads.

   b. At the top, write in the space provided the participant's name and the condition (i.e., supine).

5. Follow the appropriate post-ECG procedures.

   a. When the test period is over, press the 000 button and remove the leads from the participant's electrodes.

   b. Remove the gray cord from the electrocardiograph.

   c. Roll the cord up and put it into the drawer on the front of the cart.

   d. Turn off the power on the monitor and the electrocardiograph.

Discussion Questions

1. What are the basic dimensions and characteristics on the paper grid used for an ECG? Describe the horizontal and vertical measurements that can be taken.

2. Describe the basic components of the cardiac cycle as it is represented on an ECG.

3. Describe the 10 locations for the electrodes on a standard 12-lead electrocardiograph.

Bibliography

ACSM (American College of Sports Medicine).1993. *ACSM's Resource Manual for Guidelines for Exercise Testing and Prescription*, 2nd ed. Philadelphia: Lea & Febiger.

ACSM (American College of Sports Medicine). 2000. *ACSM's Guidelines for Exercise Testing and Prescription*, 6th ed. Baltimore: Lippincott Williams & Wilkins.

Dubin, D. 1990. *Rapid Interpretation of EKGs*, 4th ed. Tampa, FL: Cover.

PART III

Exercise Prescription

PART III focuses on exercise prescription. The initial lab in this section addresses the calculation of metabolic work for use in exercise prescription. The next two labs focus on the three phases of exercise prescription (initial, improvement, and maintenance), assessment of the participant's goals, and gaining the participant's commitment to the exercise prescription. The final lab in this manual challenges students to apply the techniques and principles presented in this laboratory manual by developing case studies. This process is facilitated by the worksheets and forms employed in earlier labs. The forms are in appendix A and the worksheets in appendix B; remember to photocopy them for use in the labs.

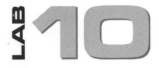
Metabolic Calculations

PURPOSE

This lab demonstrates the knowledge and skill required to determine $\dot{V}O_2$ levels at given workloads in relative and absolute measures, MET levels, and kcal expenditure.

MATERIALS

1. Calculator
2. Problems 1-10 (pages 95-97)
3. Metabolic equations in appendix E (pages 160-161)
4. % HRR and %$\dot{V}O_2$R Calculation Worksheet (page 148)

Background Information

Metabolic equations serve two purposes for exercise professionals. The first is to calculate oxygen consumption, which allows the professional to determine caloric expenditure for a specific activity and duration. The second enables the exercise professional to determine a target workload specific to the individual's goals and needs.

You can use several methods to determine target workload intensity for exercise prescription. ACSM (2000) recommends using %$\dot{V}O_2$ reserve (%$\dot{V}O_2$R) instead

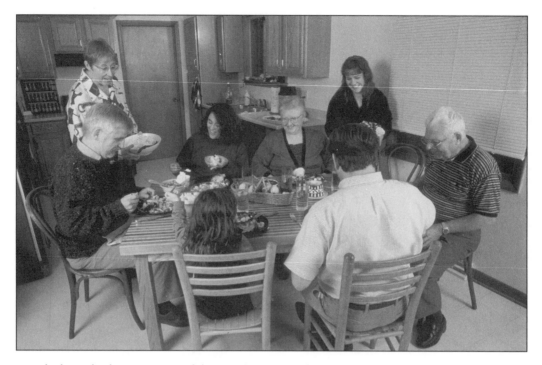

Metabolic calculations are vital for good nutritional management.

of %$\dot{V}O_2$. This is because Swain and Leutholtz (1997) demonstrated that %VO_2R corresponds with %HR reserve (%HRR) more closely than does a direct percentage of $\dot{V}O_2$max. HRR accounts for the effect of varying resting HR levels from one person to the next and the impact of resting HR (RHR) on determining exercise intensity. To calculate %HRR and %$\dot{V}O_2R$, the resting measure of these variables (RHR and 3.5 ml/kg/min, respectively) is subtracted from the maximal levels of these variables, then the target percentage is calculated from this difference, and finally the resting measure is added back. The %HRR and %$\dot{V}O_2R$ Calculation Worksheet (page 148) presents these steps clearly. The prescribed range of intensities of exercise for %HRR and %$\dot{V}O_2R$ (40-85%) is discussed in lab 11.

Procedures

Solve the following problems. You may use a calculator if necessary. You may find appendix D, Metric Conversions (pages 158-159), helpful as you complete this lab.

Problem 1

At maximal effort John Jones is running on a treadmill at 5.6 mph up a 10% grade. His current body weight is 165 lb. Calculate the following:

    a. Relative $\dot{V}O_2$ in ml/kg/min

    b. Absolute $\dot{V}O_2$ in L/min

    c. MET level

    d. kcal/min

    e. Target $\dot{V}O_2$ at 75% $\dot{V}O_2R$

Problem 2

Hamid Hoodah is walking on a treadmill at 4 mph for 45 min. His current body weight is 240 lb. His current functioning $\dot{V}O_2$ level is 2.9 L/min. Calculate the following:

    a. kcal/min

    b. Total caloric expenditure

    c. Relative $\dot{V}O_2$ in ml/kg/min

    d. MET level

    e. Grade of the treadmill

Problem 3

Keshaun Jackson is running on a treadmill at a certain speed with a grade of 7% at 42.27 ml/kg/min for 30 min. His body weight is 185 lb. Calculate the following:

    a. Absolute $\dot{V}O_2$ in L/min

    b. The speed of the treadmill

    c. MET level

    d. kcal/min

    e. Total caloric expenditure

Problem 4

Pauline Koh is cranking an arm ergometer at 50 rpm with a resistance of 2 kg. This is her maximum workload. Her body weight is 110 lb. The distance for each revolution of the resistance wheel is 2.4 m, and the number of revolutions per minute is 50. Calculate the following:

    a. Relative $\dot{V}O_2$ in ml/kg/min

    b. Absolute $\dot{V}O_2$ in L/min

    c. MET level

    d. kcal/min

    e. Target $\dot{V}O_2$ at 80% $\dot{V}O_2R$

Problem 5

Moesha Turner weighs 140 lbs and is walking up and down an 8-in. step at 30 steps/min for 45 min. Calculate the following:

    a. Relative $\dot{V}O_2$ in ml/kg/min

    b. Absolute $\dot{V}O_2$ in L/min

    c. MET level

    d. kcal/min

    e. Total caloric expenditure

Problem 6

Danielle Lowenstein's maximum workload while riding a cycle ergometer at 60 rpm is 4 kg of resistance. Her body weight is 120 lb. The distance for each revolution of the cycle ergometer is 6 m. Calculate the following:

    a. Relative $\dot{V}O_2$ in ml/kg/min

    b. Absolute $\dot{V}O_2$ in L/min

    c. MET level

    d. kcal/min

    e. Target $\dot{V}O_2$ at 65% of $\dot{V}O_2R$

Problem 7

Amit Patel is running on a treadmill at 6.7 mph at an 8% grade for 30 min. His body weight is 185 lb. Calculate the following:

    a. Relative $\dot{V}O_2$ in ml/kg/min

    b. Absolute $\dot{V}O_2$ in L/min

    c. MET level

    d. kcal/min

    e. Total caloric expenditure

Problem 8

Suki Takahashi is running on a treadmill at 6.6 mph at a 5% grade for 45 min. Her body weight is 125 lb. Calculate the following:

    a. Relative $\dot{V}O_2$ in ml/kg/min

    b. Absolute $\dot{V}O_2$ in L/min

    c. MET level

    d. kcal/min

    e. Total caloric expenditure

Problem 9

Maria Garza steps on a 15-in. step at 25 steps/min for 30 min. She weighs 125 lb. Calculate the following:

    a. Relative $\dot{V}O_2$ in ml/kg/min

    b. Absolute $\dot{V}O_2$ in L/min

    c. MET level

    d. kcal/min

    e. Total caloric expenditure

Problem 10

Angus Magnussen is walking on a treadmill at 3.6 mph for 30 min. His current body weight is 240 lb. His absolute $\dot{V}O_2$ level at this intensity is 2.9 L/min. Calculate the following:

    a. Relative $\dot{V}O_2$ in ml/kg/min

    b. MET level

    c. The grade of the treadmill

    d. kcal/min

    e. Total caloric expenditure

Bibliography

ACSM (American College of Sports Medicine). 2000. *ACSM's Guidelines for Exercise Testing and Prescription,* 6th ed. Baltimore: Lippincott Williams & Wilkins.

Swain, D.P., and B.C. Leutholtz. 1997. Heart rate reserve is equivalent to % $\dot{V}O_2$ Reserve, not % $\dot{V}O_2$ max. *Medicine and Science in Sports and Exercise* 29: 410-14.

Prescriptions for Initial Conditioning, Improvement, and Maintenance

PURPOSE

This lab presents and describes the general principles of exercise prescription. Students will learn to integrate fitness assessment results into information that they can use in prescribing exercise for their clients.

MATERIALS

1. One copy of the Fitness Assessment Form With Exercise Prescription Guidelines (page 124)
2. Three copies of the %HRR and %$\dot{V}O_2$R Calculation Worksheet (page 148)

Background Information

The ACSM guidelines for exercise prescription are based on a plethora of data that have provided evidence for the specific stimulus necessary to cause adaptations to the cardiovascular and musculoskeletal systems. These adaptations are based

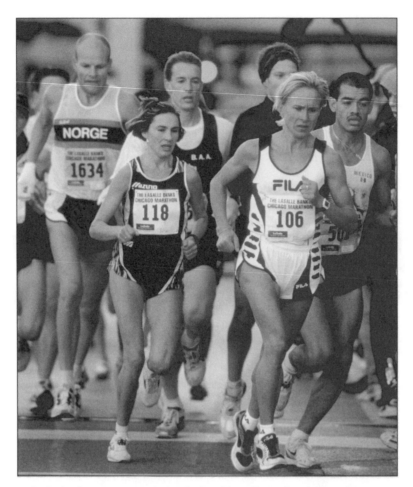

If she is so minded, almost any apparently healthy client should be able to run a marathon if you provide her with a well-designed training regimen.

on the principles of overload (repeated exposure, including appropriate rest, to unaccustomed load is associated with adaptation of improved functional capacity), specificity (adaptations are specific to stimulus and systems involved), and progression (improved functioning requires increases in stimulus to cause further adaptation) (ACSM 2000). Furthermore, the guidelines for caloric expenditure are supported with evidence demonstrating the impact of caloric expenditure on weight loss and body composition (United States Department of Health and Human Services 1996).

Training Session Components

Each training session should contain three components: warm-up phase, stimulus (exercise) phase, and cool-down phase. These phases are important in allowing the body's systems to prepare for activity and recover appropriately from activity. Most important, the cardiovascular system adapts to meet the oxygen requirements of the activity, while the musculoskeletal system adapts to facilitate movement by reducing the viscosity of joint lubricants. These adaptations may reduce the likelihood of injury. With regard to the four major components of health-related fitness, the warm-up phase or the cool-down phase can include musculoskeletal flexibility. The stimulus or exercise phase can be either a cardiorespiratory stress or a skeletal muscle stress, with energy expenditure being calculated for aerobic activity.

The ACSM exercise prescription guidelines are presented in the Fitness Assessment Form With Exercise Prescription Guidelines (page 124). These guidelines are intentionally broad and must be used with good clinical judgment based on the client's fitness level, health status, personal interests and goals, and age.

Individualizing Exercise Prescriptions

Following are factors to address when prescribing exercise.

Cardiorespiratory Fitness

HR and $\dot{V}O_2$ maintain a positive linear relationship as workload increases. This relationship allows for the determination of exercise intensity through the calculation of percentage of HR reserve (%HRR; Karvonen equation) and percent $\dot{V}O_2$ reserve (%$\dot{V}O_2$R). These two methods provide reliable and relatively accurate measures of exercise intensity. Following are the equations for %HRR and %$\dot{V}O_2$R. If calculating exercise intensity from a straight percentage of HRmax you can expect that %$\dot{V}O_2$max will be 10-15% lower than the %HRmax. Note that RPE can be a useful tool in identifying a workload that is comfortable for the client. In particular, for clients who are taking a medication that can alter HR or those who have difficulty palpitating HR, RPE can be helpful in providing a cue for determining exercise intensity (ACSM 2000; Howley and Franks 2003; Pollock et al. 1998).

Percent heart rate reserve (%HRR):

(HRmax – resting HR) × % intensity + resting HR = target HR

Percent $\dot{V}O_2$ reserve (%$\dot{V}O_2$R):

($\dot{V}O_2$max – resting $\dot{V}O_2$) × % intensity + resting $\dot{V}O_2$ = target $\dot{V}O_2$

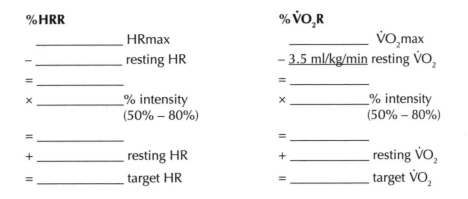

Energy Expenditure

The expenditure of energy can be a significant concern to those who are beginning an exercise program. A good understanding of how the body utilizes energy for physical activity can limit participants' unrealistic expectations about weight loss. Unrealistic expectations are also likely to impact motivation. The metabolic cost of a prescribed activity can be determined with the metabolic calculation presented in lab 10. Furthermore, this metabolic cost can be used to determine the caloric expenditure of that activity. Following is an example of the calculations for a person who weighs 75 kg.

Determining the caloric expenditure of running at 5 mph at a 2% grade using metabolic calculations yields a $\dot{V}O_2$ of 32.61 ml/kg/min (which would be a target $\dot{V}O_2$).

> 32.61 ml/kg/min –3.50 ml/kg/min (subtract 1 MET to determine net caloric expenditure); 29.11 ml/kg/min ÷1,000 (to convert to L/kg/min); .02911 L/kg/min × 75 kg (to convert to L/min); 2.18 L/min × 5 kcal/min (standard used for kcal expenditure for $\dot{V}O_2$ in L/min); 10.9 kcal/min expended

If the goal is 1,000 kcal/week, the client would have to accumulate 91.7 min of this activity throughout the week (1,000 kcal ÷ 10.9 kcal/min = 91.7). The client could achieve this caloric expenditure with approximately 30 min of this activity 3 days/week.

Musculoskeletal Flexibility

Lack of flexibility in the lower back and posterior thigh regions seems to be associated with increased risk for development of chronic low back pain. Furthermore, maintaining flexibility may facilitate elderly people's ability to perform activities of daily living. Proprioceptive neuromuscular facilitation (PNF) is not advised for use by anyone without specific knowledge of the techniques.

Muscular Fitness

People require some level of muscular strength and endurance to perform activities of daily living. Thus, maintaining muscular fitness is critical for maintaining functional independence throughout the life span and limiting musculoskeletal injury. It is important to avoid the Valsalva maneuver when lifting heavy weight; this is accomplished by expiring when moving the weight against gravity (concentric contraction) and inspiring when moving the weight with gravity (eccentric contraction).

Progression Through Exercise Prescription

Following are the guidelines for progressing through the three stages of an exercise program (ACSM 2000).

1. Initial conditioning stage
   - The initial conditioning stage should progress through 4 weeks.
   - Unfit, inactive participants should start at 40-60% of HRR.

- Each session should last 15-20 min initially and progress to 30 min.
- Schedule 3-4 sessions/week (reevaluate goals—address whether goals should be adapted for any initial adaptations that may have occurred).
- Begin a strength-training program with light weights and slowly progress to the Fitness Assessment Form With Exercise Prescription Guidelines (page 124).

2. Improvement stage
   - The improvement stage typically lasts 4-5 mo.
   - Periodically reassess fitness and reevaluate goals.
   - For most people, the target range for intensity should progress to 85% of HRR.
   - Increase duration every 2-3 weeks until the client can perform moderate-to-vigorous exercise continuously for 20-30 min.
   - Schedule 3-5 sessions/week.
   - Alter the strength-training program to facilitate the adaptations necessary to meet goals.

3. Maintenance stage
   - This stage typically begins after 5-6 mo, when the participant has reached preestablished fitness goals and is no longer interested in further increases in the conditioning stimulus.
   - The client's focus should turn to meeting long-term goals (reassess fitness and reevaluate goals).
   - The activities selected for this phase should be enjoyable and promote lifetime participation in physical activity.
   - Reevaluate strength goals and alter the strength-training program accordingly.

The exercise prescription for enhancing muscular fitness should increase in resistance as adaptations occur and goals are achieved. To maintain muscular fitness, perform at least one set of 8-10 different exercises at least twice a week.

Flexibility should be addressed throughout each stage. Following initial assessments, the prescription should focus on enhancing range of motion for the muscle groups that the client is using during the physical activity session and those that are determined to be limiting the client's range of motion. Following this initial adaptation, the prescription for flexibility should be directed toward addressing the client's goals and any limitation or misalignment that is diagnosed (Griffin 1998).

Procedures

1. Complete the Fitness Assessment Form With Exercise Prescription Guidelines (page 124) for at least one person in the class.

2. From lab 10 (metabolic calculations) determine the caloric expenditure for three of the problems. Calculate the number of 30-min workouts per week each of the three individuals in the problems would have to complete to expend 1,000 kcal.

3. Calculate %HRR for each of those three individuals.

Discussion Questions

1. What are some concerns to consider when prescribing resistance exercise?

2. As time progresses and the client is adapting to the exercise stress, what issues and factors should you address to maintain motivation and compliance?

Bibliography

ACSM (American College of Sports Medicine). 2000. *ACSM's Guidelines for Exercise Testing and Prescription.* Baltimore: Lippincott Williams, & Wilkins.

Griffin, J.C. 1998. *Client-Centered Exercise Prescription.* Champaign, IL: Human Kinetics.

Howley, E.T., and B.D. Franks. 2003. *Health Fitness Instructor's Handbook,* 4th ed. Champaign, IL: Human Kinetics.

Pollock, M.L., G.A. Gaesser, J.D. Butcher, J.P. Deprés, R.K. Dishman, B.A. Franklin, and C.E. Garber. 1998. The recommended quantity and quality of exercise for developing and maintaining cardiorespiratory and muscular fitness, and flexibility in healthy adults. *Medicine and Science in Sports Exercise* 30: 975-91.

United States Department of Health and Human Services. 1996. *Physical Activity and Health: A Report of the Surgeon General.* Washington, DC: International Medical Publishing.

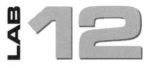
Assessing Participant Goals and Gaining Commitment to Exercise

PURPOSE

This lab facilitates exercise prescription and adherence by demonstrating how to assess the participants' fitness and health goals. As physical adaptations occur and fitness is improved, fitness and health goals may also change. Thus assessment follows a series of cyclical steps:

1. Assessment of health-related fitness
2. Modification of behavior (developing an exercise prescription to achieve goals)
3. Monitoring behavior (exercise journals, record keeping)
4. Periodic reevaluation of health-related fitness, modification of behavior (if necessary), and continual monitoring of behavior (Griffin 1998).

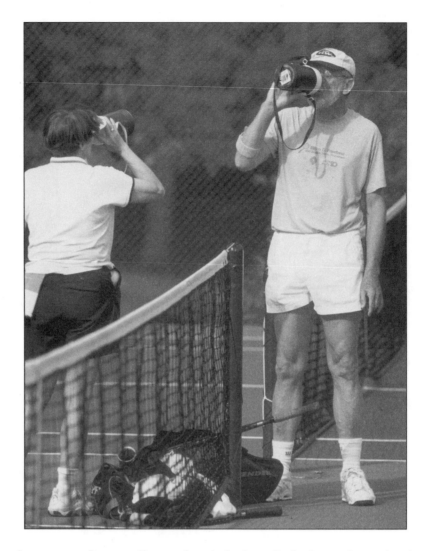

You must know your clients well enough to help them find a form of exercise they enjoy.

MATERIALS

Two copies each of the following forms:

1. Exercise Prescription Interview Form (page 126)
2. Fitness Goals and Exercise Prescription Form (page 127)
3. Fitness Contract (page 128)
4. Resistance Exercise Journal (page 129)
5. Cardiovascular Exercise Journal (page 130)

Background Information

Four steps of client motivation are integral to developing an effective exercise prescription.

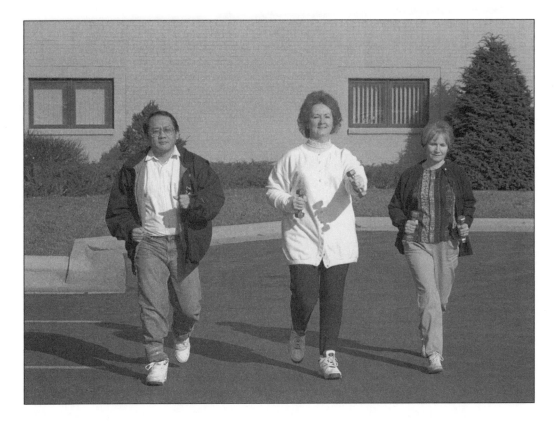

If your clients are especially busy, you must help them find activities they can fit into their busy days, such as vigorous walking during breaks at work.

1. **Assessment of health-related fitness**

   As you initiate a relationship with a client, it is important to present and conduct yourself in a professionally appropriate manner. In addition, effective motivators who enhance adherence most often have a positive rapport with clients. This can be important for maintaining open communication.

2. **Modification of behavior** (develop an exercise prescription to achieve goals)

   - Interview the client to assess his or her health-related fitness goals **(Exercise Prescription Interview Form)**.
   - Establish goals that include a clear strategy for achieving each goal. **(Fitness Goals and Exercise Prescription Form)**
     - The goals should be challenging and attainable.
     - Each goal must be desirable to the client.
     - There should be both short-term and long-term goals.
     - Goals should be highly specific and practical.
     - The client must believe that the exercise prescription created to achieve the goal will be effective.
     - The client must believe that the exercise prescription is achievable.

- With the client, fill in the "exercise prescription" areas of the Fitness Goals and Exercise Prescription Form using the guidelines from the client's Fitness Assessment Form With Exercise Prescription Guidelines that address each goal.
- Guide the client in examining and addressing both environmental support for and barriers to implementing the prescription strategies for each goal.
- Have the client rate importance, commitment, and confidence for reaching each goal. This is likely to illuminate motivation issues that you may want to address (Griffin 1998).
- Behavioral contracts (Fitness Contracts) can be used to demonstrate and document commitment to the fitness program.

3. **Monitoring of behavior** (exercise journals, record keeping)
- Clients should keep a clear daily record of the behaviors that are part of the goal strategies (Fitness Journals).

4. **Periodic reevaluation**
- Health-related fitness should continue to be the focus.
- Modification of behavior may be necessary when life events impact exercise behavior.
- Monitoring behavior can ensure that the client is continually aware of his or her exercise behaviors.

Procedures

1. Complete one set of the forms for yourself. You need to fill out only one week in the resistance and cardiovasular exercise journals.

2. Find one other person outside of class and take him or her through the process of completing the second set of forms. This person needs to complete the exercise journals for only one week.

Discussion Questions

1. What are some important characteristics of a professional in the fitness-promotion field?

2. How can an exercise specialist build rapport with a client?

3. What are factors to consider when setting goals? What should be included in a complete goal-setting program?

4. In setting goals, how might a client address expected barriers to an exercise program?

5. How would you handle a client who is having difficulty following the proposed strategy for achieving his or her goal?

6. Would you expect that goals might change as the client ages, achieves certain goals, or has a change in daily schedule? How would you handle a situation in which a client does want to change his or her goals?

Bibliography

ACSM (American College of Sports Medicine). 2000. *ACSM's Guidelines for Exercise Testing and Prescription*. Baltimore: Lippincott, Williams, & Wilkins.

Griffin, J.C. 1998. *Client-Centered Exercise Prescription*. Champaign, IL: Human Kinetics.

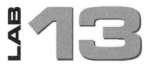

Case Study Reports

PURPOSE

This lab provides an opportunity for students to develop case studies on a variety of fitness program participants.

MATERIALS

1. Case studies from lab 3
2. Equipment for fitness testing
3. Four copies of Medical History Form (page 117) or its shorter alternative, the Health Screening Form (page 116)
4. Four copies of Informed Consent Form (page 120)
5. Four copies of Physician Release Form (if necessary) (page 121)
6. Four copies of Risk Stratification Form (page 122)
7. Four copies of Fitness Assessment Form With Exercise Prescription Guidelines (page 124)
8. Four copies of Exercise Prescription Interview Form (page 126)
9. Four copies of Fitness Goals and Exercise Prescription Form (page 127)
10. Four copies of Fitness Contract (page 128)
11. Copies of the corresponding worksheets to the data that you collected on your case studies

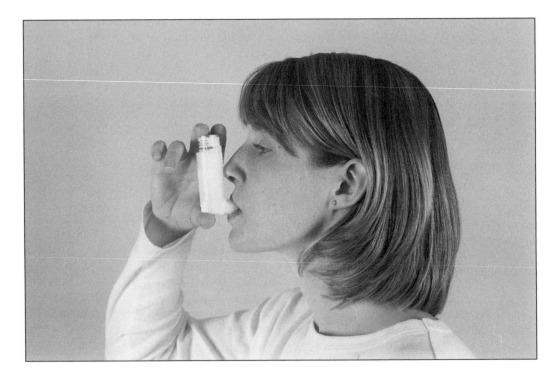

You must know your client's history in order to prescribe exercise appropriately—as with this client who has asthma.

Background Information

The prescription for exercise training must be formulated as carefully as any other preventive or therapeutic intervention. The development of an adequate and safe exercise prescription depends on the availability of the following information:

1. Sufficient medical information to assess the client's past and present health status, including patient demographics, a medical and surgical history, findings of a physical examination, signs and symptoms, essential test results (blood chemistry, ECG, echocardiography, and angiography), and a risk factor assessment and profile

2. Graded exercise test data (if advised) that quantify current physical work capacity

3. Documentation of current exercise habits

4. The client's expression of interests, needs, and objectives for wanting to participate in an exercise-training program

A case study is a concise report of the essential information pertaining to the risk status, exercise evaluation, or activity prescription of a given person. The following procedures are steps that can simplify the development of a case study using the forms presented throughout this lab manual.

Procedures

1. Review the case studies in lab 3.

2. Create four new case studies and exercise prescriptions for four classmates or volunteers. Remember to include
   a. the Medical History Form or it shorter alternative, the Health Screening Form,
   b. the Informed Consent Form,
   c. the Physician Release Form (if necessary),
   d. testing results and calculations,
   e. the Risk-Stratification Form,
   f. the Fitness Assessment Form With Exercise Prescription Guidelines,
   g. the Exercise Prescription Interview Form,
   h. the Fitness Goals and Exercise Prescription Form, and
   i. the Fitness Contract.

3. Suggest any other appropriate preventive or therapeutic interventions.

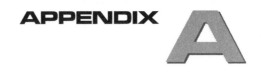

Exercise Testing and Prescription Forms

HEALTH SCREENING FORM

Name: _____ Date: _____

Male: _____ Female: _____ Age: _____ Height: _____ Weight: _____

This form is intended to obtain relevant information about your health that will assist the staff in helping you with your program. Please answer all questions to the best of your knowledge.

1. Weight

   How would you describe your current body weight?

   _____ Underweight (under ideal)   _____ 5 to 19 lb overweight

   _____ Normal   _____ More than 20 lb overweight

2. Blood pressure

   Do you have high blood pressure?   Yes   No

   Have you had high blood pressure in the past?   Yes   No

   Are you on medication for high blood pressure?   Yes   No

3. Smoking

   Do you smoke?   Yes   No

   Are you a former smoker?   Yes   No

   If yes, please give the date you quit. _____

4. Diabetes

   Do you have diabetes?   Yes   No

5. Heart problems

   Have you ever had a heart attack?   Yes   No

   Have you ever had heart surgery?   Yes   No

   Have you ever had angina?   Yes   No

6. Family history

   Have any of your blood relatives had heart disease, heart surgery, or angina?   Yes   No

7. Orthopedic problems

   Do you have any serious orthopedic problems that would prevent you
   from exercising?   Yes   No

   If yes, please explain.

   _____

   _____

   _____

8. Other problems

   Do you have any reason to believe you should not exercise?   Yes   No

   If yes, please explain.

   _____

   _____

   _____

9. Emergency

   Please list a relative we may contact in case of an emergency:

   Name: _____ Telephone: _____

   Relation: _____

From *Exercise Testing and Prescription Lab Manual* by Edmund Acevedo and Michael Starks, 2003, Champaign, IL: Human Kinetics.

MEDICAL HISTORY FORM

Name: _____ Date:_____

Address: _____ Age: _____ Date of birth: _____

_____ Sex: _____ Height: _____ Weight: _____

Home phone: (___) _____ Business phone: (___) _____

In case of emergency contact _____

Contact's phone: (___) _____

Name of personal physician: _____

Date/Reason last consulted: _____

Physician's phone: (___) _____

1. Please place a check mark beside those conditions that you currently have or have had in the past.

   _____ heart attack   _____ thrombophlebitis   _____ 5 to 19 lbs overweight
   _____ angina   _____ asthma   _____ high blood pressure
   _____ abnormal ECG   _____ fixed-rate pacemaker _____ low blood pressure
   _____ heart medications _____ embolism   _____ diabetes
   _____ valve disease   _____ respiratory infections _____ epilepsy
   _____ aneurysm   _____ irregular heartbeats _____ anemia

2. Has your physician ever advised you against exercise?   _____ Yes _____ No
   If yes, why? _____
   _____
   _____

3. Do you have or have you had any of the following conditions?

   _____ arthritis   _____ ankle/foot injury   _____ shoulder/clavicle injury
   _____ low back pain   _____ arm/elbow injury   _____ knee/thigh injury
   _____ calcium deposits _____ nerve damage   _____ upper back injury
   _____ head/neck injury _____ bone fracture   _____ wrist/hand injury
   _____ hip/pelvis injury _____ tennis elbow

   If yes, why? _____
   _____
   _____

4. Are you currently receiving physical therapy?   _____ Yes _____ No
   If yes, please furnish your therapist's name and phone number: _____
   _____   (   ) _____

5. May we call him/her?   _____ Yes _____ No

6. Do you have any conditions or past injuries that may limit the range of motion of your muscles, joints, bones, spinal column, or any other part of your body that may be aggravated by exercise?   _____ Yes _____ No
   If yes, please explain: _____
   _____
   _____

(continued)

MEDICAL HISTORY FORM (cont.)

7. Are you currently taking any medications on a regular basis? _____Yes _____ No
   If yes, please list names and dosages of each: _____
   _____
   _____

8. Are you currently under a doctor's care? _____Yes _____ No
   If yes, please furnish his/her name and phone number: _____
   _____ (___)_____

9. May we call him/her? _____Yes _____ No

10. What is your current weight? _____

11. What was your weight 1 year ago? _____ 5 years ago: _____ at age 20? _____

12. Are you currently on a specific diet? _____Yes _____ No
    If yes, please describe: _____
    _____
    _____

13. Are you tired or fatigued most of the day? _____Yes _____ No

14. Are you tired or fatigued at a specific time of the day? _____Yes _____ No
    If yes, when: _____
    _____
    _____

15. On the average, how many times per year do you travel extensively? _____

16. On the average, how many hours a day do you spend at work? _____
    How many days a week? _____

17. How would you rate the level of physical activity you perform while at work?
    _____ very inactive _____ inactive _____ moderate _____active _____very active

18. How would you rate the level of physical activity you perform during leisure time?
    _____ very inactive _____ inactive _____ moderate _____active _____very active

19. Are you presently performing any standard physical fitness program (e.g., aerobics)?
    _____Yes _____ No
    Explain: _____
    _____
    _____

20. How physically fit do you feel at present?
    _____ unfit _____ less than fit _____ fit _____more than fit _____very fit

21. Providing the equipment and facilities were available, which physical activities would you be
    interested in learning about and participating in?

_____ hiking	_____ bicycling	_____ aerobics
_____ weightlifting	_____ swimming	_____ jogging
_____ handball	_____ calisthenics	_____ volleyball
_____ tennis	_____ badminton	_____ racquetball/squash
_____ golf	_____ yoga	_____ supervised conditioning
_____ sailing	_____ horseback riding	program

(continued)

MEDICAL HISTORY FORM (cont.)

22. Do you have any exercise equipment or device at home?   _____Yes _____ No
    If yes, specify: _____
    _____
    _____

23. Did you participate in high school or college athletics?   _____Yes _____ No
    If yes, please specify: _____
    _____
    _____

24. Do you think that there are any activities that would not interest you or might cause you dis-
    comfort or pain?   _____Yes _____ No
    If yes, please specify: _____
    _____
    _____

25. What are your primary reasons for visiting _____:
    name of your facility

    _____ general conditioning   _____ swimming   _____ stress reduction
    _____ muscular strength   _____ running   _____ socializing
    _____ flexibility   _____ weight loss   _____ facility offerings
    _____ cardiovascular conditioning

I have answered the preceding questions to the best of my ability. I have understood all the questions asked of me and have been given the opportunity to have any questions clarified to my satisfaction. I further understand that thorough and honest responses to these questions are essential to my safety, health, and wellness.

Signature _____ Date _____

Witness _____ Date _____

From *Exercise Testing and Prescription Lab Manual* by Edmund Acevedo and Michael Starks, 2003, Champaign, IL: Human Kinetics.

INFORMED CONSENT FORM

1. Purpose and Explanation of the Test

The test you will perform will be on a cycle ergometer. The test will begin with a low amount of effort and will increase gradually depending on your fitness level. This increase in effort will continue until you reach your target heart rate or symptoms such as fatigue, shortness of breath, or discomfort appear. At that point, the cycle ergometer will be slowed. It is important that you understand you may stop the test at any point if you are feeling fatigue or any other discomfort.

2. Attendant Risks and Discomforts

During the exercise test a possibility of adverse changes exists. The changes can include abnormal blood pressure, fainting, disorders of heart rhythm, and in very rare instances, heart attack. A preliminary examination and observations during testing will help to minimize risks. Emergency equipment and trained personnel are available to deal with complications.

3. Responsibilities of the Participant

Knowledge you have of previous medical conditions and current health status directly affects your safety during the exercise test. It is your responsibility to fully disclose any medical conditions or physical abnormalities you may have as well as medications recently taken. This includes any unusual feeling you may perceive during the test. It is extremely important that you communicate with the testing staff.

4. Benefits to Be Expected

The results obtained from this test will be used in the evaluation of your current health status and to determine the activities that are appropriate for you.

5. Inquiries

We encourage any questions about the procedures and results of the exercise test. If you have any further questions, please ask.

6. Use of Medical Records

All information obtained from this exercise test will be treated as confidential. It will not be released or revealed to any person without your express written consent. The information gathered may be used for statistical or scientific purposes with your right of privacy retained.

7. Freedom of Consent

I give my consent freely to engage in an exercise test to ascertain my exercise capacity as well as the condition of my cardiovascular health. My permission to perform this exercise test is given willingly. I understand that I am free to stop the test at any time if I so choose.

I have read this consent form and I understand it, and any questions which may have occurred to me have been answered to my satisfaction. I consent to participate in this test.

Signed: _____   Date: _____/_____/_____

_____   _____
               Witness   Physician supervising test

From *Exercise Testing and Prescription Lab Manual* by Edmund Acevedo and Michael Starks, 2003, Champaign, IL: Human Kinetics.

PHYSICIAN RELEASE FORM

Dear Doctor:

_____ has applied for enrollment in the fitness-testing
(name of applicant)
and\or exercise programs at _____.
(name of your facility)

The fitness-testing program involves a submaximal test for cardiorespiratory fitness, body composition analysis, flexibility test, and muscular strength and endurance tests. The exercise programs are designed to start at an easy level and become progressively more difficult over time. All fitness tests and exercise programs will be administered by qualified personnel trained in conducting exercise tests and exercise programs.

By completing the following form, you are not assuming any responsibility for our administration of the fitness-testing and/or exercise programs. If you know of any medical or other reasons why the applicant's participation in the fitness-testing and/or exercise programs would be unwise, please indicate so on this form.

Report of Physician

____ I know of no reason that the applicant may not participate.

____ I believe the applicant can participate, but I urge caution because:

_____

_____

_____

____ The applicant should not engage in the following activities:

_____

_____

_____

____ I recommend that the applicant NOT participate.

Physician signature_____Date_____

Address_____Telephone_____

City and State_____Zip_____

From *Exercise Testing and Prescription Lab Manual* by Edmund Acevedo and Michael Starks, 2003, Champaign, IL: Human Kinetics.

RISK STRATIFICATION FORM

Name: _____   Date: _____

Risk factors	Yes/No	Comments
Positive (Yes +1)		
Family history	_____	_____
Cigarette smoking	_____	_____
Hypertension	_____	_____
Hypercholesterolemia	_____	_____
Impaired fasting glucose	_____	_____
Obesity	_____	_____
Sedentary lifestyle	_____	_____
Negative (Yes -1)	_____	_____
High serum HDL cholesterol	_____	_____

Total risk factors _____

Major signs or symptoms suggestive of CVD or PVD (Yes +1)	Yes/No	Comments
Pain, discomfort in the chest (or other anginal equivalent), neck, jaw, arms, or other areas that may be due to ischemia	_____	_____
Shortness of breath at rest or with mild exertion	_____	_____
Dizziness or syncope	_____	_____
Orthopnea or paroxysmal nocturnal dyspnea	_____	_____
Palpitations or tachycardia	_____	_____
Intermittent claudication	_____	_____
Known heart murmur	_____	_____
Unusual fatigue or shortness of breath with usual activities	_____	_____

Total signs or symptoms _____

(continued)

RISK STRATIFICATION FORM (cont.)

Initial risk stratification

Low risk _____   Moderate risk _____ High risk _____

Current medical examination

	Low risk	Moderate risk	High risk
Moderate exercise	**Not necessary**	**Not necessary**	**Recommended**
Vigorous exercise	**Not necessary**	**Recommended**	**Recommended**

Physician supervision of exercise test

Submaximal test	**Not necessary**	**Not necessary**	**Recommended**
Maximal test	**Not necessary**	**Recommended**	**Recommended**

Additional Medical Concerns

Medications: _____

_____

_____

_____

_____

_____

Orthopedic limitations: _____

_____

_____

_____

_____

_____

_____

Other:_____

_____

_____

_____

_____

_____

Note: For all **positive risk factors** that are answered **yes,** add 1 in the space provided, and for all **negative risk factors** answered **yes,** subtract 1 in the space provided. For all **signs or symptoms** answered **yes,** add 1 to the space provided. Scores should be totaled and the individual stratified according to ACSM guidelines.

From *Exercise Testing and Prescription Lab Manual* by Edmund Acevedo and Michael Starks, 2003, Champaign, IL: Human Kinetics.

FITNESS ASSESSMENT FORM
WITH EXERCISE PRESCRIPTION GUIDELINES

Fitness Assessment Results	Fitness Level Classification		Exercise Prescription Guidelines
	Percentile	Rating	

Cardiorespiratory fitness

$\dot{V}O_2$max _____ ml/kg/min

Mode: Large muscle group for prolonged periods of activity

Frequency: 3-5 days per week

Intensity: 40-85% of %HRR or % $\dot{V}O_2R$; RPE of 12-16

Duration: 20-30 min

Musculoskeletal flexibility

Sit-and-reach _____ in.

Shoulder elevation _____ in.

Mode: Static or Proprioceptive Neuromuscular Facilitation (PNF)

Frequency: 2-3 days per week

Intensity: Position of mild discomfort

Duration: 10-30 sec for static; 6 sec contraction followed by 10-30 sec of assisted stretch for PNF

Repetitions: 3-4 for each stretch

Muscular fitness

Upper body endurance:
_____ reps

Abdominal endurance:
_____ reps

Upper body strength:
_____ 1 RM

Leg strength:
_____ 1 RM

Mode: Resistance training (8-10 exercises)

Frequency: 2-3 days per week

Intensity: A resistance (weight) that will elicit volitional exhaustion within 8-12 reps for individuals less than 50 yr of age, and 10-15 reps for more frail or older individuals. 1-2 min between sets.

Duration: Each rep lasting approximately 2 sec for concentric and eccentric contractions (controlled manner)

Repetitions: 8-12 reps for individuals less than 50 yr of age and 10-15 reps for more frail or older individuals.

(continued)

124

FITNESS ASSESSMENT FORM
WITH EXERCISE PRESCRIPTION GUIDELINES (cont.)

Fitness Assessment Results	Fitness Level Classification		Exercise Prescription Guidelines
	Percentile	Rating	
Energy expenditure			
Body fat _____ %	_____	_____	**Caloric threshold:** 1,000 kcal per week; 150-400 kcal per day
Body mass index			
_____ kg/m²	_____ (classification)		
Waist circumference			
_____ cm	_____ (classification)		

*These results and guidelines should be presented to the client prior to the development of fitness goals and an exercise prescription.

From *Exercise Testing and Prescription Lab Manual* by Edmund Acevedo and Michael Starks, 2003, Champaign, IL: Human Kinetics.

EXERCISE PRESCRIPTION INTERVIEW FORM

Before this interview, be sure that the client is informed of the benefits and importance of fitness, his or her specific health-related fitness assessment results, and the exercise prescription guidelines. The fitness-assessment results and the exercise prescription guidelines are found on the Fitness Assessment Form With Exercise Prescription Guidelines (page 124). It is also important that the client be aware of the connection between choice of health-related behaviors and health fitness-related outcomes (e.g., improved overall health, enhanced fitness, decrease in morbidity and mortality).

Preferences and Interests Related to Fitness

What mode (type) of physical activity do you enjoy (e.g., walking, bicycling, jogging, swimming, doing yardwork, etc.)?

_____

_____

_____

_____

Do you prefer group or individual training? What type of training environment do you prefer (e.g., outdoor, indoor, cold, hot, pool, etc.)

_____

_____

_____

_____

Are there activities that you do not like and would like to avoid?

_____

_____

_____

_____

Would you like to do the same activities regularly, or would you prefer variety in your workout schedule?

_____

_____

_____

_____

Would you like more information or resources on particular activities or health-related information?

_____

_____

_____

_____

From *Exercise Testing and Prescription Lab Manual* by Edmund Acevedo and Michael Starks, 2003, Champaign, IL: Human Kinetics.

FITNESS GOALS AND EXERCISE PRESCRIPTION FORM

Be sure to set challenging, attainable, desirable, specific, and practical goals. The exercise prescription should also meet these criteria and follow the ACSM guidelines for exercise prescription. In your exercise prescription be sure to address factors that may be used to support you in reaching your goal and address possible hurdles/barriers that may deter you from reaching your goal. Be sure to rate how important reaching the goal is for you, how committed you are to the goal, and how confident you are in reaching the goal.

Fitness goal A: _____

Exercise prescription: _____

_____

_____

0	10	20	30	40	50	60	70	80	90	100

Low			*Moderate*			*High*
Importance			*Importance*			*Importance*
Commitment			*Commitment*			*Commitment*
Confidence			*Confidence*			*Confidence*

Importance score _____

Commitment score _____

Confidence score _____

Fitness goal B: _____

Exercise prescription: _____

_____

_____

0	10	20	30	40	50	60	70	80	90	100

Low			*Moderate*			*High*
Importance			*Importance*			*Importance*
Commitment			*Commitment*			*Commitment*
Confidence			*Confidence*			*Confidence*

Importance score _____

Commitment score _____

Confidence score _____

From *Exercise Testing and Prescription Lab Manual* by Edmund Acevedo and Michael Starks, 2003, Champaign, IL: Human Kinetics.

FITNESS CONTRACT

This **Fitness Contract** is made and entered into by and between _____ and _____. This contract is subject to the following terms and conditions:

1. To the best of my abilities I will follow the strategies set forth within my **Fitness Goals and Exercise Prescription**.

2. To the best of my abilities I will document my fitness related behaviors in my **Fitness Journal.**

3. As time progresses, when necessary I will refresh my commitment by reading and reviewing information related to health behaviors and health outcomes.

4. I will reassess my fitness level within 6 weeks (___/___/___). At that time I will reevaluate my **Fitness Goals** and if necessary set new goals.

In witness whereof, the parties hereto have executed this Fitness Contract on this the _____ day of _____ , 2003.

_____   _____
Fitness Client Signature   Fitness Consultant

From *Exercise Testing and Prescription Lab Manual* by Edmund Acevedo and Michael Starks, 2003, Champaign, IL: Human Kinetics.

RESISTANCE EXERCISE JOURNAL

Name: _____

Exercise	Warm-up	Working set	% 1 RM	Date	Comments
	x	x			
	x	x			
	x	x			
	x	x			
	x	x			
	x	x			
	x	x			
	x	x			
	x	x			
	x	x			
	x	x			
	x	x			
	x	x			
	x	x			
	x	x			
	x	x			
	x	x			
	x	x			
	x	x			
	x	x			
	x	x			
	x	x			
	x	x			
	x	x			
	x	x			
	x	x			
	x	x			
	x	x			
	x	x			
	x	x			
	x	x			
	x	x			
	x	x			

From *Exercise Testing and Prescription Lab Manual* by Edmund Acevedo and Michael Starks, 2003, Champaign, IL: Human Kinetics.

CARDIOVASCULAR EXERCISE JOURNAL

Week 1

Date	Activities	Time of day	HR/RPE	Comments/Notes
____	_____	_____	_____	_____
____	_____	_____	_____	_____
____	_____	_____	_____	_____
____	_____	_____	_____	_____
____	_____	_____	_____	_____
____	_____	_____	_____	_____
____	_____	_____	_____	_____
____	_____	_____	_____	_____
____	_____	_____	_____	_____
____	_____	_____	_____	_____
____	_____	_____	_____	_____
____	_____	_____	_____	_____

Week 2

Date	Activities	Time of day	HR/RPE	Comments/Notes
____	_____	_____	_____	_____
____	_____	_____	_____	_____
____	_____	_____	_____	_____
____	_____	_____	_____	_____
____	_____	_____	_____	_____
____	_____	_____	_____	_____
____	_____	_____	_____	_____
____	_____	_____	_____	_____
____	_____	_____	_____	_____
____	_____	_____	_____	_____
____	_____	_____	_____	_____
____	_____	_____	_____	_____

From *Exercise Testing and Prescription Lab Manual* by Edmund Acevedo and Michael Starks, 2003, Champaign, IL: Human Kinetics.

Data Collection Worksheets

CYCLE ERGOMETER CALIBRATION WORKSHEET

1. Make sure the bike is on a level surface.
2. Record the precalibration readings.
3. Scale reading (lb/kg)   Measured weight (lb/kg)

    1: _____   1: _____

    2: _____   2: _____

    3: _____   3: _____

    4: _____   4: _____

4. Adjust the plate to zero (no tension).
5. Calibrate the pendulum weight.
6. Record the calibrated readings.
7. Scale reading (lb/kg)   Measured weight (lb/kg)

    1: _____   1: _____

    2: _____   2: _____

    3: _____   3: _____

    4: _____   4: _____

8. Complete each linearity graph using a ruler or straightedge.

Measure   Precalibration   Measure   Calibrated

                        Scale   Scale

From *Exercise Testing and Prescription Lab Manual* by Edmund Acevedo and Michael Starks, 2003, Champaign, IL: Human Kinetics.

SPHYGMOMANOMETER/ANEROID GAUGE
CALIBRATION WORKSHEET

1. Zero out the gauges (be sure they are set to zero).
2. Inflate the instruments.

Mercury column (mmHg)

1: _____

2: _____

3: _____

4: _____

Aneroid gauge (mmHg)

1: _____

2: _____

3: _____

4: _____

3. Complete the linearity graph.

Aneroid reading

Mercury pressure

From *Exercise Testing and Prescription Lab Manual* by Edmund Acevedo and Michael Starks, 2003, Champaign, IL: Human Kinetics.

WEIGHT SCALE CALIBRATION WORKSHEET

1. Zero out the scale (be sure the weights are set to zero).
2. Place the varying weights on the scale.

Weight (lb/kg)

1: _____

2: _____

3: _____

4: _____

Scale reading (lb/kg)

1: _____

2: _____

3: _____

4: _____

3. Complete the linearity graph.

Scale reading

Weight

From *Exercise Testing and Prescription Lab Manual* by Edmund Acevedo and Michael Starks, 2003, Champaign, IL: Human Kinetics.

CHATILLON SCALE/LOAD CELL WORKSHEET

1. Disconnect the chair/harness.
2. Place the varying weights on the scale.

Scale (lb/kg)

1: _____

2: _____

3: _____

4: _____

Measured (lb/kg)

1: _____

2: _____

3: _____

4: _____

3. Complete the linearity graph.

Scale reading

|
|
|
|
|
|
|
|_____
Weight

From *Exercise Testing and Prescription Lab Manual* by Edmund Acevedo and Michael Starks, 2003, Champaign, IL: Human Kinetics.

SKINFOLD AND CIRCUMFERENCE
DATA COLLECTION WORKSHEET

Participant's name: _____   Date: ____/____/____

Skinfold Measurements

Sites in duplicate (within 1-2 mm)

  1. **Abdominal:**   _____   +   _____ / 2   =   _____

  2. **Biceps:**   _____   +   _____ / 2   =   _____

  3. **Chest:**   _____   +   _____ / 2   =   _____

  4. **Medial calf:**   _____   +   _____ / 2   =   _____

  5. **Midaxillary:**   _____   +   _____ / 2   =   _____

  6. **Subscapular:**   _____   +   _____ / 2   =   _____

  7. **Supraillium:**   _____   +   _____ / 2   =   _____

  8. **Thigh:**   _____   +   _____ / 2   =   _____

  9. **Triceps:**   _____   +   _____ / 2   =   _____

Circumferential Measurements

Sites in duplicate (within 1 cm)

  1. **Waist:**   _____   +   _____ / 2   =   _____

  2. **Hip:**   _____   +   _____ / 2   =   _____

From *Exercise Testing and Prescription Lab Manual* by Edmund Acevedo and Michael Starks, 2003, Champaign, IL: Human Kinetics.

HEART RATE AND BLOOD PRESSURE
DATA COLLECTION WORKSHEET

Participant's name: _____   Date: ____/____/____

Resting HR Measurements

Resting BP Measurements

1. 10-second count: _____ × 6 = _____bpm   BP reading: _____/_____

2. 15-second count: _____ × 4 = _____ bpm   BP reading: _____/_____

3. 30-second count: _____ × 2 = _____ bpm   BP reading: _____/_____

4. 60-second count: _____ bpm

Exercise HR and BP Measurements

Stage	Minute	HR	BP	Comments
1	1:00 2:00 3:00	____	___/___	
2	4:00 5:00 6:00	____	___/___	
3	7:00 8:00 9:00	____	___/___	
4	10:00 11:00 12:00	____	___/___	
Recovery	1:00 2:00 3:00	____ ____ ____	___/___ ___/___ ___/___	

From *Exercise Testing and Prescription Lab Manual* by Edmund Acevedo and Michael Starks, 2003, Champaign, IL: Human Kinetics.

ÅSTRAND-RYHMING
DATA COLLECTION WORKSHEET

Participant's name: _____ Date: ____/____/____

Weight: _____   Age: _____

Resting HR: _____ bpm   Resting BP: _____/_____

Exercise Data

Stage	(Time) HR	(Time) BP	RPE/Comments
1	(00:45) _____ bpm		
2	(01:45) _____ bpm	(1:30) ____/____	
3	(02:45) _____ bpm		
4	(03:45) _____ bpm	(03:30) ____/____	
5	(04:45) _____ bpm		
6	(05:45) _____ bpm	(05:30) ____/____	
	Final HR _____ bpm (average of fifth and sixth HRs)		
Recovery	(01:00) _____ bpm (02:00) _____ bpm (03:00) _____ bpm (04:00) _____ bpm	____/____ ____/____ ____/____ ____/____	

From *Exercise Testing and Prescription Lab Manual* by Edmund Acevedo and Michael Starks, 2003, Champaign, IL: Human Kinetics.

YMCA
DATA COLLECTION WORKSHEET

Participant's name: _____   Date: ____/____/____

Weight: _____   Age: _____

Resting HR: _____ bpm   Resting BP: ____/____

Age-predicted HRmax: 220 – _____ = _____ bpm

Target HR: _____ bpm (70% HR reserve or 85% of age-predicted max)

Exercise Data

Stage	(Time) HR	(Time) BP	RPE/Comments
1	(01:45) _____ bpm (02:45) _____ bpm	(2:30) ____/____	
2	(04:45) _____ bpm (05:45) _____ bpm	(5:30) ____/____	
3	(07:45) _____ bpm (08:45) _____ bpm	(8:30) ____/____	
4	(10:45) _____ bpm (11:45) _____ bpm	(11:30) ____/____	
Recovery	(01:00) _____ bpm (02:00) _____ bpm (03:00) _____ bpm (04:00) _____ bpm	____/____ ____/____ ____/____ ____/____	

From *Exercise Testing and Prescription Lab Manual* by Edmund Acevedo and Michael Starks, 2003, Champaign, IL: Human Kinetics.

YMCA V̇O₂MAX ESTIMATION GRAPH

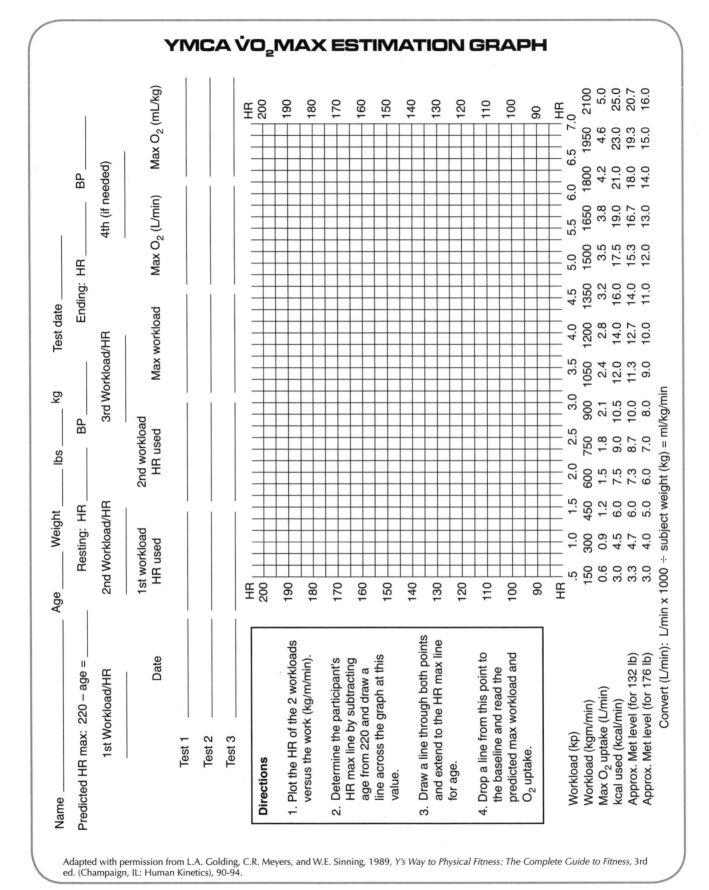

Name _____ Age _____ Weight _____ lbs _____ kg   Test date _____

Predicted HR max: 220 – age = _____   Resting: HR _____ BP _____   Ending: HR _____ BP _____

1st Workload/HR _____   2nd Workload/HR _____   3rd Workload/HR _____   4th (if needed) _____

	Date	1st workload HR used	2nd workload HR used	Max workload	Max O₂ (L/min)	Max O₂ (mL/kg)
Test 1	_____	_____	_____			
Test 2	_____	_____	_____			
Test 3	_____	_____	_____			

Directions

1. Plot the HR of the 2 workloads versus the work (kg/m/min).

2. Determine the participant's HR max line by subtracting age from 220 and draw a line across the graph at this value.

3. Draw a line through both points and extend to the HR max line for age.

4. Drop a line from this point to the baseline and read the predicted max workload and O₂ uptake.

Workload (kp)	.5	1.0	1.5	2.0	2.5	3.0	3.5	4.0	4.5	5.0	5.5	6.0	6.5	7.0
Workload (kgm/min)	150	300	450	600	750	900	1050	1200	1350	1500	1650	1800	1950	2100
Max O₂ uptake (L/min)	0.6	0.9	1.2	1.5	1.8	2.1	2.4	2.8	3.2	3.5	3.8	4.2	4.6	5.0
kcal used (kcal/min)	3.0	4.5	6.0	7.5	9.0	10.5	12.0	14.0	16.0	17.5	19.0	21.0	23.0	25.0
Approx. Met level (for 132 lb)	3.3	4.7	6.0	7.3	8.7	10.0	11.3	12.7	14.0	15.3	16.7	18.0	19.3	20.7
Approx. Met level (for 176 lb)	3.0	4.0	5.0	6.0	7.0	8.0	9.0	10.0	11.0	12.0	13.0	14.0	15.0	16.0

Convert (L/min): L/min x 1000 ÷ subject weight (kg) = ml/kg/min

Adapted with permission from L.A. Golding, C.R. Meyers, and W.E. Sinning, 1989, *Y's Way to Physical Fitness: The Complete Guide to Fitness,* 3rd ed. (Champaign, IL: Human Kinetics), 90-94.

From *Exercise Testing and Prescription Lab Manual* by Edmund Acevedo and Michael Starks, 2003, Champaign, IL: Human Kinetics.

BMI AND CIRCUMFERENTIAL SITES
DATA COLLECTION WORKSHEET AND CLASSIFICATION

BMI Calculation

Participant's name: _____   Date: ____/____/____

Calculate BMI (wt/ht^2) in the space provided.

Weight (kg): _____

Height (m): _____

BMI: _____

Classification: _____

Risk category: _____

Circumference measures

Measurement of sites in duplicate (within 1 cm)

Hip/Buttocks: _____ + _____ / 2 = _____

Waist: _____ + _____ / 2 = _____

Calculate waist-to-hip ratio in the space provided.

Risk classification: _____ (waist-to-hip ratio)

Risk classification: _____ (waist circumference)

From *Exercise Testing and Prescription Lab Manual* by Edmund Acevedo and Michael Starks, 2003, Champaign, IL: Human Kinetics.

SKINFOLD SITES
DATA COLLECTION WORKSHEET AND CLASSIFICATION

Participant's name: _____   Date: ____/____/____

Age: _____   Weight (kg): _____

Measurement of sites in duplicate (within 1-2 cm)

Calculate body fat percentage (see appendix E for formulas).

Abdominal: _____ + _____ / 2 = _____

Biceps: _____ + _____ / 2 = _____

Chest: _____ + _____ / 2 = _____

Medial calf: _____ + _____ / 2 = _____

Midaxillary: _____ + _____ / 2 = _____

Subscapular: _____ + _____ / 2 = _____

Supraillium: _____ + _____ / 2 = _____

Thigh: _____ + _____ / 2 = _____

Triceps: _____ + _____ / 2 = _____

Percentage of body fat: _____   Fat mass: _____   Lean mass: _____

Percentile: _____   Ranking: _____

From *Exercise Testing and Prescription Lab Manual* by Edmund Acevedo and Michael Starks, 2003, Champaign, IL: Human Kinetics.

MUSCULAR FITNESS
DATA COLLECTION WORKSHEET AND CLASSIFICATION

One-Repetition Maximum (1 RM) for Bench Press

Male

Participant's name: _____

Weight: _____ lb

Age: _____

____ 1 RM ÷ ____ Body weight (lb) = ____ Ratio

Percentile: _____   Rating: _____

Female

Participant's name: _____

Weight: _____ lb

Age: _____

____ 1 RM ÷ ____ Body weight (lb) = ____ Ratio

Percentile: _____   Rating: _____

1 RM for Leg Press

Male

Participant's name: _____

Weight: _____ lb

Age: _____

____ 1 RM ÷ _____ BW = _____ Ratio

Percentile: _____   Rating: _____

Female

Participant's name: _____

Weight: _____ lb

Age: _____

____ 1 RM ÷ ____ BW = _____ Ratio

Percentile: _____   Rating: _____

One-Minute Curl-Up (Crunch) Endurance

Male

Participant's name: _____

Age: _____

# of reps: _____

Percentile: _____   Rating: _____

Female

Participant's name: _____

Age: _____

# of reps: _____

Percentile: _____   Rating: _____

(continued)

MUSCULAR FITNESS
DATA COLLECTION WORKSHEET AND CLASSIFICATION
(cont.)

One-Minute Push-Up Endurance

Male

Participant's name: _____

Age: _____

# of reps: _____

Percentile: _____   Rating: _____

Female

Participant's name: _____

Age: _____

# of reps: _____

Percentile: _____   Rating: _____

Grip Strength

Male

Participant's name: _____

Age: _____

Dominant hand (kg): _____

Percentile: _____   Rating: _____

Female

Participant's name: _____

Age: _____

Dominant hand (kg): _____

Percentile: _____   Rating: _____

From *Exercise Testing and Prescription Lab Manual* by Edmund Acevedo and Michael Starks, 2003, Champaign, IL: Human Kinetics.

FLEXIBILITY DATA COLLECTION WORKSHEET AND CLASSIFICATION

Ankle Flexibility Test

Male

Participant's name: _____

Left ankle

_____ degrees dorsiflexion of best trial

-_____ degrees plantar flexion of best trial

=_____ degrees flexibility

Percentile: _____   Rating: _____

Right ankle

_____ degrees dorsiflexion of best trial

-_____ degrees plantar flexion of best trial

=_____ degrees flexibility

Percentile: _____   Rating: _____

Female

Participant's name: _____

Left ankle

_____ degrees dorsiflexion of best trial

-_____ degrees plantar flexion of best trial

=_____ degrees flexibility

Percentile: _____   Rating: _____

Right ankle

_____ degrees dorsiflexion of best trial

-_____ degrees plantar flexion of best trial

=_____ degrees flexibility

Percentile: _____   Rating: _____

Shoulder Elevation Test

Male

Participant's name: _____

_____ Best trial × 100 ÷ _____ Arm length = _____ Shoulder elevation score

Percentile: _____   Rating: _____

Female

Participant's name: _____

_____ Best trial × 100 ÷ _____ Arm length = _____ Shoulder elevation score

Percentile: _____   Rating: _____

(continued)

FLEXIBILITY DATA COLLECTION WORKSHEET AND CLASSIFICATION (cont.)

Trunk Extension Test

Male

Participant's name: _____

_____ Best trial × 100 ÷ _____ Trunk length = _____ Trunk extension score

Percentile: _____   Rating: _____

Female

Participant's name: _____

_____ Best trial × 100 ÷ _____ Trunk length = _____ Trunk extension score

Percentile: _____   Rating: _____

Sit-and-Reach Test

Male

Participant's name: _____

Trial 1: _____   Trial 2: _____   Trial 3: _____   Best trial: _____

Percentile: _____   Rating: _____

Female

Participant's name: _____

Trial 1: _____   Trial 2: _____   Trial 3: _____   Best trial: _____

Percentile: _____   Rating: _____

(continued)

FLEXIBILITY DATA COLLECTION WORKSHEET
AND CLASSIFICATION (cont.)

Thomas Test

Participant's name: _____

Right leg hip flexors: _____ Flexible _____ Inflexible

Left leg hip flexors: _____ Flexible _____ Inflexible

Straight-Leg-Raise Test

Participant's name: _____

Right leg hip extensors: _____ Degrees of flexion; _____ Acceptable _____ Unacceptable

Left leg hip extensors: _____ Degrees of flexion; _____ Acceptable _____ Unacceptable

From *Exercise Testing and Prescription Lab Manual* by Edmund Acevedo and Michael Starks, 2003, Champaign, IL: Human Kinetics.

%HRR AND %V̇O₂R CALCULATION WORKSHEET

Percent heart rate reserve: (HRmax − Resting HR) × % Intensity + Resting HR = Target HR

Percent $\dot{V}O_2$ reserve: ($\dot{V}O_2$max − Resting $\dot{V}O_2$) × % Intensity + Resting $\dot{V}O_2$ = Target $\dot{V}O_2$

%HRR

_____ HRmax

-_____ Resting HR

= _____

× _____ % Intensity (50-80%)

= _____

+ _____ Resting HR

= _____ Target HR

% $\dot{V}O_2$R

_____ $\dot{V}O_2$max

- _3.5 ml/kg/min_ Resting $\dot{V}O_2$

= _____

× _____ % Intensity (50-80%)

= _____

+ _____ Resting $\dot{V}O_2$

= _____ Target $\dot{V}O_2$

From *Exercise Testing and Prescription Lab Manual* by Edmund Acevedo and Michael Starks, 2003, Champaign, IL: Human Kinetics.

Pharmacological Effects on Cardiorespiratory Responses to Exercise

MEDICATIONS

Nitrates

Common Drugs

Generic name	*Brand name*
Isosorbid dinitrate	Isordil®
Pentaerythritol textranitrate	Peritrate
Erythrityl tetranitrate	Cardilate®
Nitroglycerin	Nitro-bid®

Treatment

Angina pectoris (used with beta-blocker or calcium channel blocker to reduce workload).

Mechanism

Nitrates relax the smooth muscle of blood vessels by a direct effect, causing vasodilation. Decreased venous return causes decreased preload; arterial dilation decreases vascular resistance and arterial blood pressure.

Effect at Rest

Increased heart rate, decreased blood pressure, decreased workload and O_2 consumption of heart.

Effect During Exercise

Increased heart rate, decreased blood pressure, increased anginal threshold, increased exercise capacity, but decreased arterial pressure may result in hypotension.

Adaptation for Exercise Prescription

Use of medication prior to reduce anginal occurrence. Longer for cool-down in postexercise period to reduce possibility of postural hypotension. Prescription involving target heart rate needs no alteration.

Beta-Blocking Agents

Common Drugs

Generic name	Brand name
Propranolol	Inderal®
Metoprolol	Lopressor®
Nadolol	Corgard®
Atenolol	Tenormin®
Pindolol	Visken®
Timilolol	Blocadren®

Treatment

Angina pectoris, hypertension, previous MI patients, arrhythmias, migraine headaches.

Mechanism

Molecules of drug attach to beta-receptor sites of sympathetic nervous system throughout body, blocking catecholamines from attaching to sites. Some cardioselective agents act primarily on beta-2 receptors in the heart (relaxation of vascular and smooth muscle), whereas others have more agonist activity, stimulating rather than blocking receptors. (Beta-1 moderates cardiac stimulation.) Decreases heart's oxygen demands (myocardial oxygen consumption) and therefore workload by a slowing of the heart and decrease in contractility and blood pressure. May delay onset of the ischemic response.

Effect at Rest

Decreased HR, BP, and arrhythmias; pindolol does not affect resting hemodynamics.

Effect During Exercise

Increased exercise capacity in patients with angina, decreased exercise capacity in patients without angina, decreased exercise ischemia, decreased HR and BP. $\dot{V}O_2$max not affected.

Adaptation for Exercise Prescription

Addition or withdrawal of beta-blocker to the therapeutic regimen of a patient necessitates a new graded exercise test. Relationship between %$\dot{V}O_2R$ and % of HRR not altered; therefore, usual methods to calculate THR for exercise prescription are still acceptable. HRmax and training HR will be lower in persons receiving beta-blockers. Use HRmax with beta-blocker therapy.

Calcium Channel Blockers

Common Drugs

Generic name	Brand name
Verapamil	Isoptin®
Nifedipine	Procardia XL®
Diltiazem	Cardizem®

Treatment

Angina pectoris, coronary artery spasm, arrhythmias, hypertension.

Mechanism

Inhibits inward flow of calcium into cardiac and vascular smooth muscle, so calcium cannot pull troponin off actin to expose active site for crossbridge of myosin. Results in potent vasodilation, which increases coronary blood flow and supply and decreases slow-channel conductance of cardiac impulses. Affects strength of contraction.

Effect at Rest

Decreased HR (except for nifedipine/Procardia) and decreased BP.

Effect During Exercise

Same as rest; may increase exercise capacity. Normal ischemic response generally not blunted. Agents (except nifedipine) prolong the PR interval (delay the electrical conduction through the atrioventricular mode in the heart), with few other ECG effects.

Adaptation for Exercise Prescription

Addition or withdrawal of a calcium blocker to the therapeutic regimen of patient necessitates a new graded exercise test. Exercise prescription should be calculated by using data from an exercise test performed with the patient following the usual medical regimen.

Digitalis

Common Drugs

Generic name	Brand name
Digoxin	Lanoxin®
Digitoxin	Crystodigin®
Digitalis	Digitortis

Treatment

Congestive heart failure (CHF), atrial fibrillation, atrial flutter.

Mechanism

Improves myocardial contraction by altering the calcium utilization of the myocardial cell.

Effect at Rest

No significant change in HR, BP, or exercise capacity, except for a decrease in HR due to vagal effect.

Effect During Exercise

May decrease HR; will improve exercise capacity only in patients with atrial fibrillation or chronic heart failure (CHF). May produce false-positive results on the ECG, or ST segment depression in patients without coronary artery disease or ischemia. Use should be stopped 10 to 14 days prior to exercise test if possible.

Diuretics

Common Drugs

Generic name	*Brand name*
Furosemide	Lasix®, Furoside
Triamterene	Dyazide®
Chlorothiazide	Diuril®
Spironolactone	Aldactone™

Treatment

Hypertension, edema (swelling—cardiac, renal, hepatic).

Mechanism

Most diuretics alter renal function, resulting in increased excretion of electrolytes and fluid by the following means:

1. Benzothiazides inhibit reabsorption of sodium and chloride in the distal tubule.
2. Loop diuretics inhibit sodium and chloride reabsorption in the ascending loop of Henle.
3. Potassium-sparing diuretics are antagonist of aldosterone, or inhibit sodium reabsorption and potassium excretion.

Reduction of blood pressure and venous return in those with hypertension, reduced workload on heart, therefore, reduced O_2 demand.

Effect at Rest

No effect on HR; may decrease BP.

Effect During Exercise

May decrease BP; may affect CHF patient, may induce arrhythmias (PVCs due to hypokalemia). HR or exercise capacity is typically not affected; however, hypovolemia may result in decreases in cardiac output, renal perfusion, and blood pressure.

Adaptation for Exercise Prescription

Check for hypokalemic conditions in patients receiving diuretics. Hypotension possible in postexercise period caused by hypovolemia; avoid dehydration before and after exercise; increase cool-down period.

Vasodilators

Common Drugs

Generic name	*Brand name*
Hydralazine	Apresoline®
Minoxidil	Loniten®
Captopril	Capoten®

Treatment

Hypertension, CHF.

Mechanism

Hydralazine and minoxidil act directly on vascular smooth muscle to cause relaxation and dilation. Captopril inhibits angiotensin-converting enzyme (ACE), which indirectly results in vasodilation (inhibits conversion of AI to vasoconstrictor AII). This vasodilation reduces blood pressure (decreases afterload). Results in decreased blood pressure and workload of the heart. Undesirable effects include increased HR and contractility, which impose a greater workload on the heart.

Effect at Rest

Decrease in BP, possible increase in HR.

Effect During Exercise

Reflex tachycardia, which may bring on anginal response. Postexercise hypotension may be accentuated by any of these meds.

Adaptation for Exercise Prescription

Gradual cool-down for prevention of hypotension after exercise. Effects of meds on Exercise Prescription are related to their effects on HR. Exercise Prescription should be based on exercise test results while medicated.

Sympatholytics (Drugs Interfering With SNS)

Common Drugs

Generic name	Brand name
Reserpine	Serpasil
Guanethidine	Ismelin
Propranolol	Inderal®
Alpha-methyldopa	Aldomet®
Prazosin	Minipress®

Treatment

Treatment of hypertension.

Mechanism

Variety of mechanisms, but all agents interfere with the effects of the SNS on the blood vessels and/or the heart by depleting or preventing the release of NE, reducing HR and contractility, decreasing activity of the SNS in the brain, or blocking alpha receptors in the vessels causing vasodilatation.

Effect at Rest

May decrease resting HR; decreases resting BP. Reserpine may cause depression, fatigue, and decreased desire for exercise.

Effect During Exercise

May decrease HR; decreases BP. No effect noted on ECG or exercise capacity.

Adaptation for Exercise Prescription

Some medications may produce orthostatic hypotension, especially immediately after exercise. Gradual cool-down recommended.

Anticoagulant Agents

Common Drugs

Generic name	Brand name
Sodium Heparin	Hepathrom, Lipo-hepin
Bishydroxycoumarin	Dicumarol, Liquaemin Sodium Warfarin Coumadin®

Treatment

Thromboembolic conditions

1. Myocardial infarction
2. Rheumatic heart disease
3. Cerebrovascular disease

Mechanism

Heparin inactivates thrombin and therefore prevents conversion of fibrinogen to fibrin.

Coumarin inhibits synthesis of the vitamin K–dependent clotting factors.

Adaptation for Exercise Prescription

Does not seem to interfere with graded exercise testing.

Anti-Lipidemic Agents

Common Drugs

Generic name	Brand name
Nicotinic Acid	Nicobid®, Nicolar®, Slo-Niacin®, Niaspan®
Clofibrate	Artomid-S
Cholestyrimine	Cuemid, Questram
Probucol	Lorelco
Colestipol	Colestic
Gemfibrozil	Lopid®
Atorvastatin	Lipitor®
Fluvastatin	Lescol®
Lovastatin	Mevacor®

Treatment

Reduction of elevated serum lipids to reduce morbidity and mortality in atherosclerosis and coronary artery disease.

Mechanism

Reduces serum or plasma cholesterol.

Effect at Rest

With some exceptions, these agents have no effect on HR, BP, or ECG.

Effect During Exercise

These agents would not affect exercise tolerance in any direct fashion and would not interfere with graded exercise testing.

Anti-Arrhythmic Agents

Common Drugs

Generic name	Brand name
Digoxin	Lanoxin®
Diphenylhydantoin	Dilantin®
Lidocaine	Xylocaine®
Procainamide	Pronestyl®
Propranolol	Inderal®
Quinidine	Cardioquin®
Disopyramide	Norpace®
Verapamil	Isoptin®

Treatment

Regulate abnormal cardiac rhythms.

Mechanism

All anti-arrhythmics are utilized to normalize rhythm disturbances through diverse mechanisms.

1. Norpace: Decreases NA conductance, reduce conduction velocity
2. Dilantin: Increases K conductance, decreases conduction velocity and depressed NA conductance in ischemic tissues
3. Inderal: Produces beta-adrenergic receptor blockage
4. Isoptin: Blocks calcium channel activity

Effect at Rest

Reestablishes normal heart rhythm, which results in more efficient functioning, which results in reduced demand for oxygen. Resting values can be varied.

Effect During Exercise

By restoring a normal sinus rhythm, anti-arrhythmics improve exercise tolerance by allowing the heart to function more efficiently. Each of the classes of drugs will also modify the ECG.

Adaptation for Exercise Prescription

Exercise test for purpose of exercise prescription need not be performed because these agents do not significantly affect HR, but it is recommended that these drugs be used at time of test due to their effect on cardiac rhythm.

Psychotropic Agents

Common Drugs

Generic name	Brand name
(major tranquilizer)	
phenothiazine	Thorazine®, Mellaril®

Treatment

Prescribe antipsychotic medications, major tranquilizers.

Mechanism

Anticholinergic and direct myocardial depressant alpha-adrenergic blockade

Effect at Rest

May result in elevated HR, decreased BP, orthostatic hypertension. The following ECG changes occur: increased PR and QT intervals (electrical conduction abnormalities), QRS widening, ST segment depression, blunting of T-wave.

Tricyclic Antidepressants

Common Drugs

Generic name	Brand name
Imipramine, Amitriptyline	Tofranil®, Elavil®
Desipramine	Norpramin®

Treatment

Prescribe antidepressant.

Mechanism

Block intake of NE in CNS.

Effect at Rest

May have increased HR, lower BP, increased tendency for arrhythmias, orthostatic hypotension, inversion or flattening of T-wave, possible false-positive test results.

Anti-Anxiety Agents

Common Drugs

Generic name	Brand name
Meprobamate	Miltown®, Equanil®
Chlordiazepoxide	Librium®
Diazepam	Valium®

Treatment

Prescribe anti-anxiety agent.

Mechanisms

Vary

Effect at Rest

Mild hypotension, no significant effects on hemodynamics or ECG findings, with exception of possible lowering of HR and BP.

Effect During Exercise

No effect on exercise capacity.

Other Agents

Alcohol

1. Depresses heart indirectly by acting within the CNS.
2. Recent studies show chronic excessive use has a deleterious effect on the heart (may produce myocardial damage).

3. Not a coronary vasodilator.
4. Alcohol may prevent the sensation of anginal pain, probably due to central depressant effects.
5. Alcohol will not suppress the ECG changes that occur with exercise testing in patients with coronary atherosclerosis, but it may suppress associated anginal pain.

Thyroid Meds

1. When used to correct thyroid abnormality, and maintain state of euthyroidism, no abnormal cardiovascular effects.
2. Levothyroxine (Synthrox)—may produce elevations of HR and BP at rest and during exercise; cardiac arrhythmias, possible ischemia and angina

Cold Remedies

1. Phenylpropanolamine, phenylephrine, pseudoephedrine
2. These agents may transiently increase HR and BP

Nicotine

1. Ganglionic stimulant
   a. Vasoconstriction, elevated blood pressure
   b. Tachycardia
   c. a. and b. result in increased cardiac workload
   d. Because of release of epinephrine and NE, resulting effects include increases in HR and SBP, DBP, and pulse pressures
   e. Excessive use may cause
      - premature systole;
      - atrial tachycardia;
      - decrease in amplitude and inversion of T-wave; or
      - angina and myocardial ischemia, atrial or ventricular arrhythmias.

Broncodilators/Antihistamines

Common Drugs

Generic name	Brand name
Aminophylline	Btheo-Dur
Isopropterenol	Bisuprel
Theophylline	

Treatment

Asthma, chronic obstructive pulmonary disease (COPD)

Mechanism

Inhibit bronchial smooth-muscle constriction in patients with asthma or COPD.

Effect at Rest

May increase HR; may produce arrhythmia; BP effect will vary.

Effect During Exercise

May increase HR; may increase BP; may produce PVCs and dysrhythmias. Increases exercise capacity in patients limited by bronchospasms. Antihistamines: No effects on hemodynamic variables, the findings of resting or exercise ECG's, or exercise capacity.

Metric Conversions

Length Conversions

1 m = 39.370 in. = 3.281 ft = 1.0936 yd
1 cm = 0.3937 in.
1 mm = 0.03937 in.
1 km = 0.62137 mile

1 in. = 2.54 cm = 25.4 mm = 0.0254 m
1 ft = 0.3048 m
1 yd = 0.914 m = 91.44 cm
1 mile = 1609.35 m = 1.609 km

Mass (M) or Weight (Wt) Conversions

1 kg = 1 kp = 2.2046 lb
1 g = 0.0022 lb = 0.0352 oz
1 lb = 453.59 g = 0.454 kg
1 oz = 28.349 g
1 grain = 65 mg

Force (F) Conversion

1 kg = 9.80665 N
1 N = 0.10197 kg = 0.2248 lb

Volumn (V) Conversions

1 L = 1.0567 US qt (1 US qt and 1 US gal
   are >1 Imperial qt and gal)
1 US qt = 0.9464 L
1 US gal = 3.785 L
1 cup liquid = 250 ml
1 tablespoon = 15 ml

Work (w) and Energy (E) Conversions

1 Nm = 1 J = 0.7375 ft-lb
1 kgm = 9.80665 J = 7.2307 ft-lb
1 ft-lb = 0.1383 kgm = 1.3560 Nm
1 kJ = 0.239 kcal
1 kcal = 4186 J = 4.186 kJ
1 kcal = 426.85 kgm at 100% efficiency
1 J = 0.10197 kgm

1 liter of oxygen used in burning glycogen
   (respiratory quotient = 1.0)
   = 5.0047 kcals
   = 15,575 ft-lbs
   = 2153 kgm $\cdot$ min^{-1}

Velocity (v) Conversions

1 m $\cdot$ s^{-1} = 2.2371 mph
1 m $\cdot$ min^{-1} = 0.03728 mph
1 km $\cdot$ h^{-1} (kmh) = 0.6215 mph
1 mph = 26.8 m $\cdot$ min^{-1}

Radial Velocity Conversions

1 rad $\cdot$ s^{-1} = 57.3° $\cdot$ s^{-1}
rad = radian = 0.5 Π = radius of circle
   = 57.3°
1° = 0.01745 radian
Π = 3.1416 = ratio of the circumference
   of a circle to its diameter.

Power (P) Conversions

1 W = 1 J $\cdot$ s^{-1} = 60 J $\cdot$ min^{-1} = 0.060 kJ $\cdot$ min^{-1} = 6.12 kgm $\cdot$ min^{-1} = 0.1019 kgm $\cdot$ s^{-1}

1 kW = 1000 W = 1.34 hp

1 kgm $\cdot$ min^{-1} = 0.1635 W = 0.000219 hp

1 hp = 745.7 W = 745.7 J $\cdot$ s^{-1} = 75 kgm $\cdot$ s^{-1} = 4562 kgm $\cdot$ min^{-1} = 10.688 kcal $\cdot$ min^{-1}

Acceleration (a) Conversion

a of gravity = 9.81 m $\cdot$ s^{2} = 32.2 ft $\cdot$ s^{2}

Temperature (T) Conversions

each °C = 1°K = 1.8 °F

each °F = 0.56°C = 0.56°K

Pressure Units, Symbols, and Conversions

1 Pascal (Pa) = 1 N $\cdot$ m^{2}

Barometric pressure (PB): 1 in. = 25.4 torr; 29.92 in. Hg = 760 torr = 1 atm = 14.7 lb/in.

1 mbar = 0.750 mm Hg = 0.750 torr

Metabolic and Anthropometric Equations

Metabolic Equations

Walking

This formula is suitable for speeds of 50 to 100 m/min (1.9 to 3.7 mph).

$$\dot{V}O_2 = 0.1 \text{ (speed)} + 1.8 \text{ (speed)(fractional grade)} + 3.5 \text{ ml/kg/min}$$

Running

This formula is suitable for speeds of 80 to over 134 m/min (3.0 to 5.0 mph) if the participant is jogging or running.

$$\dot{V}O_2 = 0.2 \text{ (speed)} + 0.9 \text{ (speed)(fractional grade)} + 3.5 \text{ ml/kg/min}$$

Leg Ergometry

These formulas are suitable for power outputs between 50 and 200 Watts (300 – 1,200 kg/m/min).

$$\dot{V}O_2 = 1.8 \text{ (work rate)} \cdot M^{-1} + 7 \text{ ml/kg/min}$$

or

$$\dot{V}O_2 = \frac{1.8 \text{ (work rate)}}{M} + 7 \text{ ml/kg/min}$$

Arm Ergometry

These formulas are suitable for power outputs between 25 and 125 Watts (150-750 kg/m/min).

$$\dot{V}O_2 = 3 \text{ (work rate)} \cdot M^{-1} + 3.5 \text{ ml/kg/min}$$

or

$$\dot{V}O_2 = \frac{3 \text{ (work rate)}}{M} + 3.5 \text{ ml/kg/min}$$

Stepping

This formula is suitable for stepping rates between 12 and 30 steps/min, and step height between 0.04 and 0.40 m (1.6-15.7 in.).

$$\dot{V}O_2 = 0.2 \text{ (stepping rate)} + 1.33 \cdot 1.8 \text{ (step height) (stepping rate)} + 3.5 \text{ ml/kg/min}$$

Bibliography

ACSM (American College of Sports Medicine). 2000. *Guidelines for Exercise Testing and Prescription*. Baltimore: Lippincott, Williams & Wilkins.

Anthropometric Equations

Skinfold Formulas for Determining Body Density

Jackson-Pollock 7-site formula for men (chest, midaxillary, triceps, subscapular, abdomen, suprailiac, and thigh):

Body density = 1.112 − 0.00043499 (sum of 7 skinfolds) + 0.00000055 (sum of 7 skinfolds)^2 − 0.00028826 (age)

Jackson-Pollock 3-site formula for men (chest, abdomen, and thigh):

Body density = 1.10938 − 0.0008267 (sum of 3 skinfolds) + 0.0000016 (sum of 3 skinfolds)^2 − 0.0002574 (age)

Jackson-Pollock 3-site formula for men (chest, triceps, and subscapular):

Body density = 1.1125025 − 0.0013125 (sum of 3 skinfolds) + 0.0000055 (sum of 3 skinfolds)^2 − 0.000244 (age)

Jackson-Pollock 7-site formula for women (chest, midaxillary, triceps, subscapular, abdomen, suprailiac, and thigh):

Body density = 1.097 − 0.00046971 (sum of 7 skinfolds) + 0.00000056 (sum of 7 skinfolds)^2 − 0.00012828 (age)

Jackson-Pollock 3-site formula for women (triceps, suprailiac, and thigh):

Body density = 1.099421 − 0.0009929 (sum of 3 skinfolds) + 0.0000023 (sum of 3 skinfolds)^2 − 0.0001392 (age)

Jackson-Pollock 3-site formula for women (triceps, suprailiac, and abdomen):

Body density = 1.089733 − 0.0009245 (sum of 3 skinfolds) + 0.0000025 (sum of 3 skinfolds)^2 − 0.0000979 (age)

Body Density to Body Fat Conversion Formulas

Brozek body density conversion formula:

$$\frac{457}{\text{body density}} - 414.2 = \%\text{ body fat}$$

Siri body density conversion formula:

$$\frac{495}{\text{body density}} - 450 = \%\text{ body fat}$$

Determining Goal Body Fat Percentage and Target Weight

The following method can be used to determine goal body fat percentage (GBF%) and target weight (TW):

1. Multiply total body weight (TBW) by the body fat percentage (BF%) to determine fat weight (FW).
2. Subtract FW from TBW.
3. The remaining weight is the lean mass weight (LMW).
4. Determine an appropriate and reasonable GBF%.
5. Divide the LMW by the GBF% – 1.
6. The answer will be the TW at the predetermined GBF%.
7. Subtract TW from TBW to determine the amount of weight loss (WL) required to achieve GBF%.

Step-by-Step Instructions

Step 1	TBW × BF% = FW
Step 2	TBW – FW = LMW
Step 3	LMW/(GBF% – 1) = TW
Step 4	TBW – TW = WL

Bibliography

Brozek, J., F. Grande, J. Anderson, and A. Keys. 1963. Densitometric analysis of body composition: Revision of some quantitative assumptions. *Annals of the New York Academy of Science* 110: 113-40.

Jackson, A.S., and M.L. Pollock. 1985. Practical assessment of body composition. *Physician and Sports Medicine* 13: 76-90.

Siri, W.E. 1956. Body composition from fluid spaces and density: Analysis of methods. In *Techniques for Measuring Body Composition,* edited by J. Brozek and A Henshel. Washington, DC: National Academy of Sciences-National Research Council.

Glossary

aneurysm—A bulging of the wall of a blood vessel, usually caused by hardening of the arteries and high blood pressure.

angina—A symptom of some diseases that is characterized by a feeling of choking, suffocation, or crushing pressure and pain.

artifact—A distortion that does not reflect a true waveform found within electrocardiography. Often caused by excessive lead wire motion or improper electrode placement.

body composition—The percentage of body weight that is fat (% body fat) compared to total lean mass.

Chatillon scale—A hanging weight scale.

claudication—Pain of the legs consisting of cramps in the calves caused by poor circulation of blood in the legs.

dynamometer—An instrument that operates on the compression principle and is used to indicate the force required to move a needle a certain distance.

electrocardiograph (ECG)—A device that records the electric activity of the heart to detect abnormal electric impulses through the muscle.

embolism—A defect in which a clot (embolus) travels through the bloodstream and becomes lodged in a blood vessel, usually in the heart, lungs, or brain.

ergometer—An instrument used to measure the amount of work done by an organism.

ergometry—A method of measuring the amount of work done by an organism, usually during exertion.

flexibility—The ability to move the body parts through a wide range of motion.

goniometer—A protractor type of instrument used to measure the total degrees of rotation of a joint.

Gulick tape—A flexible measuring tape equipped with a spring-loaded attachment at the end that, when pulled out to a specified mark, exerts a fixed amount of tension on the tape.

isokinetic training—Training that has both variable resistance and a speed-governing feature. Because isokinetic equipment controls the rate of contraction, it can potentially train the different types of muscle fibers.

isometric contraction—A static muscle contraction wherein the overall length of the muscle does not change during the application of force against a fixed object.

isotonic contraction—A dynamic muscle contraction in which the force remains constant. Isotonic exercises are typically performed with free weights or machines in which the resistance is "steered" along a fixed path. Accommodating resistance training (e.g., Nautilus, Cybex, etc.) is considered isotonic, although resistance is variable so that the lifter must exert maximum effort throughout the full range of motion.

Karotkoff—Five phases of varying sounds heard through auscultation during blood pressure assessment.

linearity—The maximum percentage of error between the expected value and the actual sensor reading, compared to the range.

maximal oxygen consumption—The highest amount of oxygen a person can take in and utilize to produce adenosine triphosphate aerobically during heavy exercise.

muscular endurance—The ability of a muscle to exert a submaximal force over a length of time.

muscular strength—The maximum amount of force that a muscle can exert in a single maximal effort.

one-repetition maximum (1 RM)—The maximum weight that a person can lift successfully for one repetition.

random error—An error that is a result of pure chance.

scale—An instrument used to measure gross body weight.

skinfold calipers—A pincer device that measures the thickness of a double layer of finger-pinched skin and subcutaneous fat.

sphygmomanometer—An instrument made up of a rubber bladder, gauge, and rubber inflation/deflation bulb and valve that is used to measure systolic and diastolic blood pressure.

stadiometer—An instrument used to measure standing height.

stethoscope—An instrument made up of an amplification bell, a Y-shaped rubber tubing, and earpieces used to detect sounds produced by the human body.

systematic error—A predictable error systematically influenced by something other than what you are attempting to measure.

Valsalva maneuver—"Increased pressure in the abdominal and thoracic cavities caused by breath holding and extreme effort" (Howley and Franks 2003). Performing a Valsalva maneuver can inhibit the return of blood to the heart and increase blood pressure.

$\dot{V}O_2$—The rate at which oxygen is being transported to and used by the active working tissues of the body.

$\dot{V}O_2$**max**—The maximal rate at which oxygen can be transported to and used by the working tissues of the body. The most accepted index of cardiorespiratory work.

$\dot{V}O_2$ **reserve ($\dot{V}O_2R$)**—The difference between $\dot{V}O_2$max and resting $\dot{V}O_2$.

About the Authors

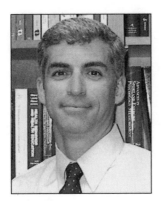

Edmund O. Acevedo, PhD, is an associate professor at the University of Mississippi, where he teaches exercise testing and prescription and serves as director of the Applied Physiology Laboratory.

Formerly a corporate fitness program coordinator, he is a fellow of the ACSM and a certified exercise specialist. His 14 years of teaching experience serve him well in the field, as do his memberships in the American Physiological Society, AAPHERD, AAASP, and NASPSPA.

Acevedo makes his home in Oxford, Mississippi, with his wife, Tracy. In his free time, he enjoys running and competing in triathlons.

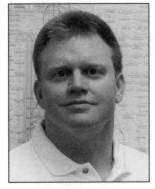

Michael A. Starks is a PhD candidate in exercise science and a graduate research and teaching assistant at the University of Mississippi. He holds a master's degree in exercise science from the University of Memphis, where he formerly served as health and fitness director of the Employee Wellness Unit.

Starks earned a graduate research fellowship at the University of Mississippi in 2001. Today he is a strength and conditioning specialist certified by the National Strength and Conditioning Association and is a CPR and first aid instructor for the National Safety Council and American Red Cross.

Starks makes his home in Oxford, Mississippi, where he enjoys resistance training and spending time with his children.